Table of Contents

Departments

2	**The Lucky Ones** by Randall J. Strossen, Ph.D.
4	**Letters to the Editor**
62	**Iron Filings** by Randall J. Strossen, Ph.D.
69	**Captains of Crush® Grippers: Who's New**
71	**Red Nail Roster**
87	**Calendar**
127	**The Iron Mine**

People

7	**Al Feuerbach: Evolutionary Thrower** by Thom Van Vleck

Training

14	**Dip, Grip, and Rip!** By Pavel
20	**Foundations: Speed, the Missing Piece of the Strength Training Puzzle** by Jon Bruney
22	**Organic Food and the Strength Athlete** by Gabriel Josiah
41	**A Great New Way to Increase Your Bench** by John Christy
46	**Pulling Sleds Made Easy** by Ernest Roy, PT, DPT
55	**Sumo Strength** by Ken Best
78	**Building a High School Weightlifting Program: Success at Sac High** by Paul Doherty
88	**The Single-Hand Deadlift** by Roger Davis
94	**Making Weight: The Forgotten Discipline** by Bill Starr
102	**Strength Skills: Lifting Hard and Heavy** by Dr. Ken E. Leistner
108	**Develop Brute Strength** by Steve Justa
123	**Advanced Shock and Variable Method: Compounding to Maximize Explosive Power–Endurance** by Steven Helmicki
125	**Working on a Training Bag** by Col. (Ret.) Joseph H. Wolfenberger

Contests

27	**2009 Arnold Weightlifting IronMind® Invitational: The Arnold Experience and Weightlifting Diplomacy** by Randall J. Strossen, Ph.D.
73	**2009 Arnold Arm Wrestling Challenge: Tough Matches at the Top Tournament** by Denise Wattles
110	**2009 European Men's Weightlifting Championships: Newcomers Make Names for Themselves** by Per Mattingsdal

History

48	**Russian Men of Might: General-Lieutenant V. G. Kostenetsky** by Joseph Svub
106	**The Very Swiss Giant: Ludwig Lutz** by Gherardo Bonini

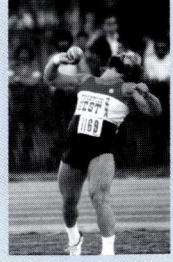

Showing his consistency and his durability, in 1978 Al Feuerbach won his fourth U.S. National Outdoor Championships and in 1979 he was the runner-up. Harry Johnson "was the coach/administrator of the first-ever Nike sponsored Track & Field Club—Athletics West, of which I was a member starting in 1977," Al explained. "Harry was not a photographer by trade, but tried to provide a service to his Athletics West athletes by capturing some of their competition moments. I visited with Harry this past summer at the 1980 Olympic Team Reunion at the 2008 Olympic Trials."
Harry Johnson photo, courtesy of Al Feuerbach.

The Lucky Ones

Anyone who's been a *MILO* reader or an IronMind customer for even a short while probably knows that we're big on hard work—not just because it's what produces results, but also because we think there's some inherent value in it.

The results thing is pretty simple and it's what the overload principle—something like the gravitational constant in the strength world—is all about: do more than you did yesterday; in fact, do more than you [easily] can if you want to gain. At IronMind, we're on record as saying that we think some people have gotten carried away with the dangers of overtraining and have underestimated the drawbacks of undertraining. Of course, most people are smart enough to avoid exertion if they can so it's no wonder that training less intensively, under whatever banner, will always be a popular theme.

We, on the other hand, chuckle as we watch the Bulgarian national weightlifting team being lectured by Ivan Abadjiev: the lifters are so exhausted that some are leaning on each other, dazed with fatigue. Abadjiev's words are stern, exhorting the lifters to do better, to lift more, or to suffer the consequences of their failure. "That's all, you are free to go," he says with a pause. "We'll start again in 15 minutes."

That's not everyday training for everyman, so we're not espousing it as a universal approach, but we can't help but admire the drive embodied by this philosophy. We also recall the time when there was a near mutiny in the Bulgarian weightlifting ranks due to the multiple 100% workouts each day. The battle lines were not drawn over the merits of this general idea, but rather over the question of whether *three* maximum-effort workouts per day were essential or whether *two* would do the trick!

There *are* limits and bodies *do* break down when pushed too hard, but all of this is merely setting the stage, giving a quick introduction to the whys and hows of hard training.

If you've ever noticed someone happily humming or whistling while working and other people who are glum when doing very little, it's apparent that the dividing line between joy and misery does not occur at the boundary of activity and rest, or even between physical comfort and discomfort in more general sense. Consider the person sitting comfortably in his nice warm car feeling grumpy, versus a soggy runner absolutely enjoying the day and his time in it.

Seek joy in your training is our advice—rather pulpit-like in its tone, but elemental in its importance, understanding that this doesn't mean you should train rarely or lightly or stick with only what you're good at. No, it means that you have to come to embrace the process, not just the results. Get busy and start to think about how lucky you are the next time you practically blow your eyeballs out of your head trying to pull a deadlift or you're an hour or two into a run and the good part is yet to come.

You're lucky enough because you're able-bodied and can do these things, and despite (because of?) your effort required, they pay you rich dividends. But you're especially fortunate because while most people never test their boundaries, you know where you are and your bonus is that you just keep getting better.

Randall J. Strossen, Ph.D.
Publisher & Editor-in-chief

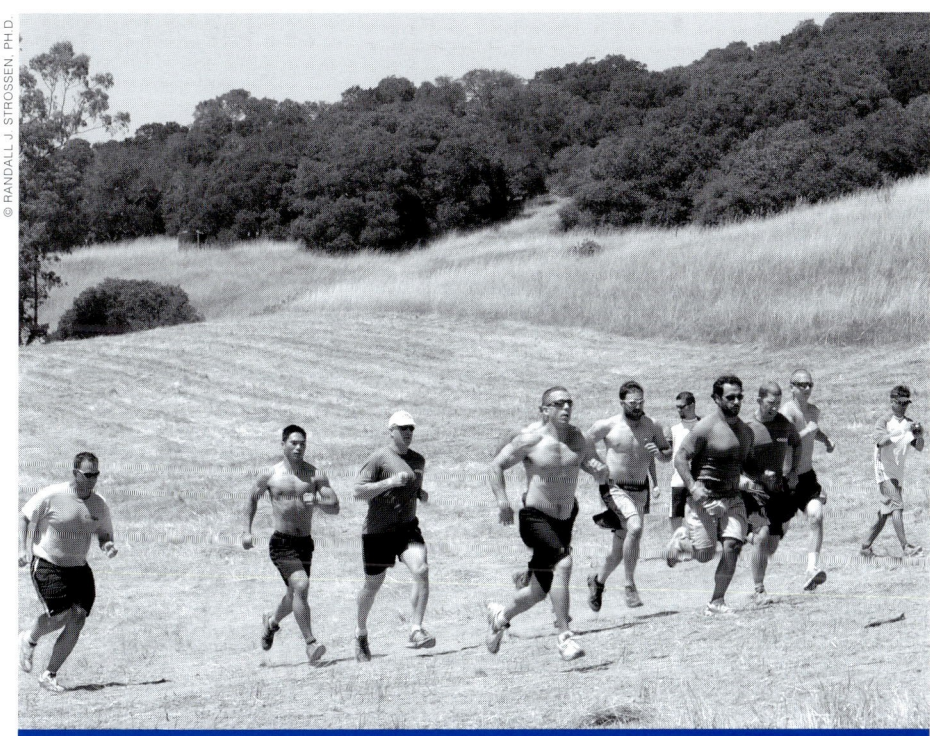

Hitting the hill at the 2008 CrossFit Games . . . proof that given a choice, not everyone runs from lactic acid build-up.
Randall J. Strossen photo.

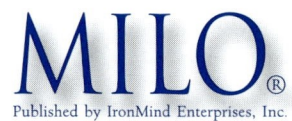

Published by IronMind Enterprises, Inc.

Randall J. Strossen, Ph.D.
Publisher & Editor-in-chief

Elizabeth M. Hammond
Production Editor

P.O. Box 1228
Nevada City, CA 95959 USA
www.ironmind.com
Tel: (530) 272-3579
Fax: (530) 272-3095
E-mail: sales@ironmind.com

MILO is published quarterly:
March, June, September &
December
Subscription rates for
4 books are:
Softcover: US$79.95/year USA;
US$89.95/year Canada/Mexico;
US$99.95/year all others
On-line:
US$39.95/year all subscribers

Single issues are:
US$20.00 each + $5.00 S&H USA
(US$7.00 S&H Canada/Mexico;
US$13.00 S&H all others)

Copyright ©2009
IronMind Enterprises, Inc.

All rights reserved.
No part of this publication
may be reproduced
or transmitted in any form
or by any means without prior
written permission except
in the case of brief quotations
embodied in articles
and reviews.

Design:
Tony Agpoon
Sausalito, CA

Letters to the Editor

Million Dollar Words

Just a follow-up to the June 2008 issue [Vol. 16, No. 1] and Steve Justa's article about core strength: I think about his comments every time I see one of my neighbors getting in their car to go the local pump and primp health club to work on their core strength. Meanwhile they pay some guy to shovel the snow in the driveway, rake the leaves, spread mulch, etc. I just came in from shoveling 6 inches of wet snow and then busted up 1-1/2 inches of ice on the driveway. Don't tell me about core exercises. I was looking forward to 20-rep squats after two hours of this. Save the expensive health club fee and the $200 "look-at-me" workout clothes and forget about paying some guy to shovel. You can do some of the best core stuff right at home and save money to buy a subscription to MILO. Just my two cents' worth.

Jeff Bates
Columbus, OH

Harness Hero

The March 2009 issue of MILO was as usual well done, including the World's Strongest Man report. The most interesting to me was the article on Paul Trappen ["World Champion of Burden Lifting: Paul Trappen" by Gherardo Bonini] whose lift of choice was the harness lift. Paul lifted 5,226 lb. in this manner, a remarkable feat on his part. At age 75-1/2, I did 1,152 lb., quite a load.

Lee Gesbeck
Fort Myers, FL

Good Stuff

I just read your intro to the March 2009 MILO ["Tough Times Aren't All Bad"] and had to shoot you a quick Bravo! You capture all the timeless and general principles that govern success under and away from the squat bar. But you also specifically point me back to my first encounter with *SUPER SQUATS* (1993) and the metaphysical and transformative effects it had on me—body, soul and spirit! As Jim "The California Cool Cat" McGoldrick would say, "Good stuff!"

Steve Jeck
Plantation, FL

Where Else But the Arnold?

I would like to thank Randall Strossen for bringing the German lifters to this year's

Arnold. We [my husband and I] have gone for the past six years as we live just north of Columbus, and every time Randy brings something special to enjoy and to be amazed at. I personally love the strength athletics, especially the strongman competition, and this did not disappoint either: Poundstone was amazing, and with Savickas out this year, everyone had a chance at the title.

I never tire of standing beside the expo stage and watching all the action; in fact it's my favorite place to be. The lifters in waiting stand right there in front of you, some of their family with them. It's a very personal experience and you want each man and woman on that stage to make their lift—it's almost impossible to pick a favorite. And the opportunities are always surprising: I was invited by a nice young man to train as a strongwoman with the Slaters (he saw me lift the log in the ASC booth)! Where else would you have something like that happen to you?

I am already counting down the days until next year. I'm sure it will be just as incredible as this year was.

Aniko Miller
Ashley, OH

MILO Connection

Although I've never met you in person, Dr. Strossen, I feel I'm a friend through the pages of *MILO*. You've done a great job bringing the best to us in training knowledge and diversity, but especially honesty. Times are hard now and I hope we can all pull through and be stronger for it. With your help through *MILO*, I know I will! Thanks.

Richard Garrett
Antioch, IL

No Dumbbell, Here

Kudos to Pavel for his excellent article on overspeed eccentric kettlebell swings "Beyond Plyometrics," March 2009, Vol. 16, No. 4).

Now that Kenneth Jay has given us "permission to go light," according to Mark Reifkind, may I suggest that we also get "permission" to use dumbbells rather than kettlebells for this particular exercise? You can do the very same overspeed eccentric swings with dumbbells without the inevitable palm damage caused by the rotating handle of a cast iron kettlebell and the painful forearm banging that can come from high-rep fatigue and ensuing deteriorating form.

I find the kettlebell a very useful tool, but to save your hands and forearms while performing the more than 500–700 swing/snatch reps involved with Jay's overspeed eccentric swing workouts, don't be a dumbbell—try one.

Steven Milloy
Potomac, MD

Setting the Record Straight

In "The Pullover and Press/Push" by Roger Davis, March 2009, Vol. 16, No. 4, page 40, Bert Burtslof is noted as doing a 215 pullover and press of 215 at 110 kg bwt. Although the lift is noted in the IAWA records, it appeared to be incorrect since the same number is listed for the pullover and push (also page 40), and generally the push result is greater than the press. Roger Davis notes on further checking with the IAWA: "It looks probably that the 215 pullover and press is an error in the 110-kg class and should belong to Larry Silvestri at 150.5 kg bwt. I actually witnessed him perform this lift in Philadelphia in 2005."

Roger also pointed out that David Gentle's article "A History of the Bench Press" [*MILO*, April 1996, Vol. 4, No. 1] credits Bill Lilley with a 220-kg pullover and push at middleweight.

Lifting That's Fun

Now here you go again, conjuring up youthful memories with your [March 2009] articles, "The Pullover and Press/Push" by Roger Davis and "The World Champion of Burden Lifting: Paul Trappen" by Gherardo Bonini (one-arm lifts).

The old York training course had some of those lifts in it, and my mentor Carl Magnuson wanted me to practice the pullover and press/push and wrestling bridge exercises for both freestyle wrestling (then called catch-as-catch-can wrestling) and hand balancing. Our acts before club organizations and shows at the YMCA included my (the 17–18-year-old) performing the one-hand deadlift (up to 315 lb.) and teeth lifting (with the same weight), and my being lifted up off the floor so Carl could spin me around while hanging by my teeth (no additional weights added).

As for the floor pullover and press, it was usually with a plate-loaded barbell, obviously lighter weights being used for the wrestler's bridge. Detroit's Belle Isle Park spectators loved watching us on the grass lawns during the summer months because we lifted weights, wrestled, and did hand balancing all day long on Saturdays and Sundays.

A gym in Detroit, Yacos, had a stage set of globe barbells. There were three—small, medium, and large. George Yacos had me as his shill at a few of his "shows" or club shindigs: he would ask me to be a part of a demonstration. Usually he would introduce me as a young weightlifter who could lift and press a heavy barbell. I would start off with the large one after George would tell the audience that I had "warmed up to it in the back."

After I would lift it and perform about 5 presses, he would then ask if any men in the audience "would like to try and outlift this young man?" Usually a couple or three men would come up and George would ask them, in order to avoid getting hurt, to start with the small barbell first. The men would try but could not get it to their shoulders. They obviously didn't try to lift the two larger barbells.

The kicker here was the small barbell with its thick handle weighed 220 lb., the middle one weighed 180 lb., and the large one weighed 120 lb. I would receive a nice ovation for my "very strong lifting." I guess I was really a fake "strong boy" but I loved it.

You may remember at the first Titan Games in San Jose (2003) when I mentioned to you about "when weightlifting was fun." Those strength lifts were fun. It is no wonder that the huge, powerful behemoths are having fun in the World's Strongest Man events. Certainly the spectators must be thrilled to see the fun WSM competitions. I really like reading about them and looking at the photos. Thank you both again for your great MILO journal.

Don Wilson
Alameda, CA

Editor's Note: We are always honored to receive a note from Don Wilson. Don and his wife Joan are longstanding fixtures at local weightlifting and Highland Games competitions, and track and field events. To read more about the Wilsons, see MILO, December 2003, Vol. 11, No. 3: "Officials Extraordinaire, Don and Joan Wilson" by Jim Schmitz.

Al Feuerbach:
Evolutionary Thrower

Thom Van Vleck
All photos courtesy of Al Feuerbach.

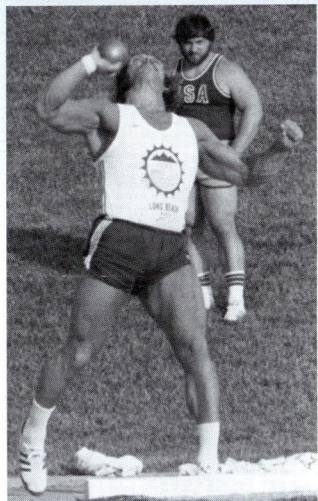

Al Feuerbach in competition.

Recently I enjoyed a road trip to one of my favorite gyms in the country, Big Al's Dino Gym in Holland, Kansas. Al Myers and I were going through a workout together and having the usual conversations about training. Being involved in Scottish Highland Games heavy events, as Al and I are, means that your heroes are often great weightlifters or great throwers. It was during this conversation that Al brought up a man who bridges that gap quite nicely, Al Feuerbach.

Al Myers competed as a pro Highland Games thrower and held the pro-class sheaf toss record at one time and was a real student of the strength game. I have always enjoyed talking to Al because he knows his stuff and I always walk away with new knowledge and inspiration. I had asked Al who his favorite thrower of all time was. You know, one of those questions to keep the conversation rolling in the right direction. Al didn't hesitate and said, "Al Feuerbach."

Al Myers said, "When I was a kid I idolized Al Feuerbach as a thrower. Sure, Randy Matson and Brian Oldfield are the big names, but I wasn't 6' 6" and neither was Feuerbach. He was a master technician who squeezed every ounce of potential out of his body. Plus, he was just a Midwestern kid like me and he went to school at Emporia State right here in Kansas. Most of all, he was a world-record holder in the shot and a national champ in Olympic-style weightlifting; he was the best in two sports."

I had, of course, heard of Al Feuerbach, and probably could have answered some basic questions about him, but I have to admit I grew up idolizing Matson and Oldfield in the shot because they were the giants; and while I'm not 6' 6", I'm close enough that I wanted to emulate the giants. Again, I walked away from the Dino Gym with more knowledge and inspiration. I wanted to learn more about Al Feuerbach, and this involved contacting the man himself.

MILO | Jun. 2009, Vol. 17, No. 1   **7**

Al Feuerbach was born in Preston, Iowa, not far from where I grew up in Missouri. He had four brothers who were all great athletes and participated in several sports. Growing up in a small Midwestern rural town in the 50s and 60s meant not much entertainment and so Al and his brothers threw themselves into sports. Al enjoyed baseball the most, but also played basketball and football and was involved in track. Al was inspired by his brother Gary, who was the first Feuerbach medalist in the Iowa State Championships in the shot put—but not the last. All five brothers were eventually Iowa State medalists in the shot put. Later, Al and his younger brother Bob would hold the world record for combined distance by brothers. His brother Tom was a decathlete of merit, and Steve was all-state in football and basketball. Gary was a baseball and basketball player. Al's dad was an athlete in his own right. He was a starter on the Iowa State basketball team in college. Sports were just a way of life. Al told me that his mother and father were very involved parents. He could not recall their missing a single sporting event in which he or his brothers competed. Al calculated this to be about 80 seasons of sports!

Al's parents instilled a strong work ethic in their children. They worked hard on the farm. Al's dad credits one particular job to Al's success: bucking bales. Stacking hay bales often involved throwing the bales, and as the stacks got higher, Al had to get creative in how he got them to the top; he frequently used a "shot-put" style to drive the bales to the top row. Al doesn't necessarily believe bucking bales made him a world-record shot putter, but he does believe the hard work ethic he learned from it was the foundation for his later success.

Al's first interest was not throwing, but weightlifting—until one day (when Al was in the 8th grade) when his older brother brought home a 12-lb. shot and left it in the back yard after a throwing session. Al picked it up and threw it and he was intrigued. He said he walked out, picked it up again and tried to throw it farther. At that moment, he was hooked for life.

Al told me, "You can actually see the improvement. With weights you know if you will set a PR or not, based on the weight on the bar. With throwing you are never quite sure." Al talked about the thrill of stretching the tape out and the anticipation of a bigger throw to come—his joy in it was evident.

> . . . HE WALKED OUT, PICKED IT UP AGAIN AND TRIED TO THROW IT FARTHER. AT THAT MOMENT, HE WAS HOOKED FOR LIFE.

Al started using a 5-lb. plate for a discus. After basketball, baseball, football—whatever the season was—he would go home and throw. There might be snow on the ground, but he would simply just go and throw over and over again. This was always after other practices—and sometimes in defiance of his coaches who worried that he was over-training. Al said, "I threw often. You have to have the mental capacity to throw that often with intensity without burning out. I loved the challenge so much, I never burned out." Al would throw two, sometimes three sessions a day. His training was often intuitive and he would try many different things. One thing he really enjoyed doing was throwing a 20-lb. shot for height to work on getting lower and getting his hips and legs into the throw. Al threw

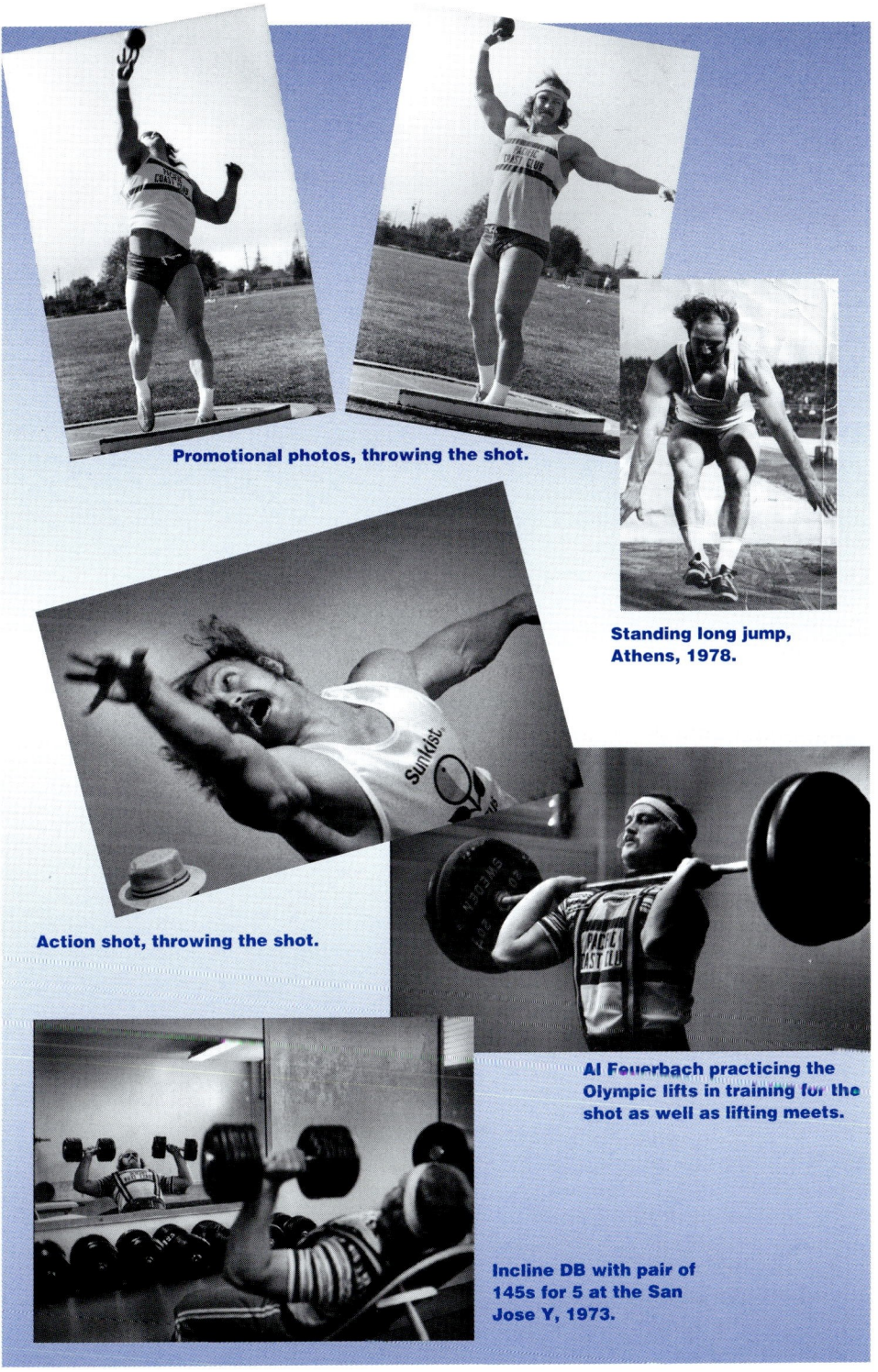

Promotional photos, throwing the shot.

Standing long jump, Athens, 1978.

Action shot, throwing the shot.

Al Feuerbach practicing the Olympic lifts in training for the shot as well as lifting meets.

Incline DB with pair of 145s for 5 at the San Jose Y, 1973.

early and often and almost every day. Al realizes he became known as a technician in order to overcome his size, but he never really thought in those terms: he just focused on throwing far and using whatever leverages were available.

Al told me that while the mind is not really a muscle, it has to be trained like the most important muscle in the body. The thought of throwing was never far from the forefront of his mind. His technique developed in an evolutionary way. As he would throw, he would analyze each throw and adapt the technique to his body. He couldn't change his leverages, so why not enhance them and throw in the way that best took advantage of his leverages. One thing that came out of this was what Al called the "pre-torque power position." Al utilized the glide styles on the shot put and he would swivel his right foot 90 degrees into the throw. This move didn't happen by design. It happened as a result of dealing with what he had available and changing his technique to put his body in the best possible position to throw.

Mental rehearsal was a big part of Al's training. He called it day dreaming, but I could see some people calling it obsessing. If you have ever been bitten by the throwing or lifting bug, you will be able to relate. Al said that while a student at Emporia State, he would think so much about throwing that he would often be unable to shut off his mind and get to sleep, so he would sometimes just get up and go train in the middle of the night. He had a key to the gym and he would go down and lift weights or he would throw in the dark.

> **THE THOUGHT OF THROWING WAS NEVER FAR FROM THE FOREFRONT OF HIS MIND.**

Al threw in a time of epic throwers. Randy Matson was just past his peak when Al came along; Brian Oldfield was rarely able to beat him head-to-head. Al mentioned that George Woods was actually his top competitor during his peak years, which lasted from 1970 to 1980. Woods was an incredible athlete who started out as a pole-vaulter and at 310 lb. could do a front flip. Woods competed in three Olympic Games and won two silver medals, missing gold by one centimeter.

When I asked Al who he thought was the greatest shot putter of all time, he initially mentioned Parry O'Brien. I thought maybe it was because Parry broke the world record 17 times, or because he was the first person to throw the 16-lb. shot more than 60', or that he won 116 consecutive competitions, but it was because Parry innovated the sport with his glide: he advanced throwing technique by using a full glide, later named the O'Brien technique. Parry threw in an evolutionary way, as Al would do later.

When pressed, Al said that he thought Randy Matson was the greatest of all time. At 6' 8", Randy was an incredible athlete, a fine technician, and the first to throw 70'. I'll mention that the second man ever to throw 70' was Al Feuerbach and that Al consistently beat Matson later in Matson's career.

That connection goes even further. Al stated that his greatest single moment was a night at the San Francisco Cow Palace in 1971. He was a relative unknown coming out of Emporia State, having just moved to California the summer before. Randy Matson was in top form and had tied the world indoor record the week before in Los Angeles. At that meet, Al was only 1.5" behind Randy, but he got no due for his effort and seethed about it all week. This led to an explosion in the Cow Palace with a throw of 68' 11" that was a new indoor world record; and he beat Matson, whom he considers to be the greatest of all time. Al had done it basically coming out of nowhere. He was called the "mod-style Kansan" and he recalled that Howard Cosell said on *Wide World of Sports*, "He may have mod hair but tonight he set an indoor world record." Al said that after all the countless hours doing field work back in Iowa and day dreaming about being on top, and then to have it happen was a very happy moment.

Al considered the Olympic lifts to be his secret weapon. In a 1971 *Sports Illustrated* interview right after Al beat Matson (as *SI* put it, "defeated the undefeatable Randy Matson") for the first time, he stated that the bench press was the most important lift in his training. He also said that every 10 lb. he put on his bench seemed to translate into 1' of distance in his throws. Al admits that this was "totally misleading information, as I didn't want a specimen the likes of Randy Matson to become aware of the importance of Olympic lifts." Al said that while he often utilized heavy dumbbell inclines, he didn't even use the bench press in his training.

> AT THAT MEET, AL WAS ONLY 1.5" BEHIND RANDY, BUT HE GOT NO DUE FOR HIS EFFORT AND SEETHED ABOUT IT ALL WEEK.

In 1973 Al Feuerbach flew from San Francisco to Moscow, Russia, to compete in a shot put meet as the only western male. It was an extraordinarily long flight, especially in the days of the Iron Curtain. Al went over 70' at that meet and then on the way back stopped off at the U.S. Weightlifting Championships to compete. After the long trip, Al went to weigh in and weighed only 241 lb.; he needed to weigh 242 lb. to compete where he wanted to, in the super heavyweight class. He spent the next hour drinking water and when he weighed in, he palmed his large watch and made weight by a fraction. He ended up in second place to Jacob Stefan. Had Al stayed at 241 lb., his total of 342.5 kg would have won the 242-lb. class and beat the legendary Bob Bednarski (whom Al had admired as a great Olympic lifter). The next year, 1974, Al went five for five attempts and won the 242-lb. class. His total of 340 kg would have beaten Bruce Wilhelm, who competed in the super heavyweight class, since that same total would have tied him for first place and he would have won on bodyweight.

Regardless, Al was not selected for the U.S. team to go the Worlds. He figured it had to do with the fact that he was perceived as a shot-putter first and would forgo the weightlifting Worlds for the shot-putting Worlds. Al stated he later caught some flak for not going; this bothered him, as he was more than willing to go but nobody asked him until it was too late for him to make

> ". . . AS I DIDN'T WANT A SPECIMEN THE LIKES OF RANDY MATSON TO BECOME AWARE OF THE IMPORTANCE OF OLYMPIC LIFTS."

the arrangements—a miscommunication that may have cost the U.S. a medal!

Al Feuerbach talked about the two-year span from 1973 to 1974 as being a special time for him. During that period he was the top-ranked shot-putter in the world, and on May 5, 1973, he set the world record in the shot at 71' 7". In 1973 he was the runner-up in the U.S. Weightlifting Nationals, and in 1974 Al won the 242-lb. class. During an 82-day span in 1974, he competed in and won 29 competitions and averaged 69' with the 16-lb. shot. Al commented that it was just "a great feeling to be in that type of competitive shape."

I asked Al for some stories that may or may not be well-known from his years in competition. Al told me about a trip to Europe in 1974. The U.S. team stopped over in West Germany to have a dual meet with the West German team. He said that four members, including Dwight Stones (19-time national high jump champion, 3-time world-record holder, and winner of two Olympic bronze medals), Steve Williams (world-record holder at the time in the 100-meter dash), and Ron Semkiw (shot-putter on the team) and himself, went on a tour of the Puma factory. On the way back they got caught in a traffic jam and missed the team bus so they grabbed a train but forgot their passports in the rush. At one point, a German police officer came by and asked for their passports and when he found out they didn't have them he said, "NO passport, off the train." Realizing they could be dropped off in the middle of nowhere and miss the meet—and that there was a real language barrier—they pulled out their uniforms, to no avail. Ron pointed out Steve was the world-record holder in the 100 meter—no effect. Next was Dwight Stones—no influence. But when he mentioned Al Feuerbach, the officer smiled and said, "Feuerbach! . . . show me muscle" in a thick German accent. Al flexed his arm and the officer nodded and said, "Ahhh, that good passport" and let them stay on the train.

Al never specifically trained on jumping for competition but in Athens, Greece, in the late 1970s, Al went over 11' in the standing long jump in an official competition. He credits doing the Olympic lifts and throwing the shot with developing his jumping ability without actually practicing jumping. He also believes it lends credence to the idea that athletes involved in Olympic lifting and throwing are among the most explosive and coordinated athletes in the world.

> HE CREDITS DOING THE OLYMPIC LIFTS AND THROWING THE SHOT WITH DEVELOPING HIS JUMPING ABILITY WITHOUT ACTUALLY PRACTICING JUMPING.

Al said that he competed in a track meet in Edinburgh, Scotland, and after the meet they donned kilts and competed with several other throwers in the Scottish Highland Games heavy events. The athletes included Geoff Capes, whom Al knew had some experience in the Games. Capes helped him through the events as Al had no experience with them whatsoever. He recalls that he did well on the weight-over-bar and the stone put, but he was proudest of picking a huge caber. He recalled there was an athlete from New Zealand who, when asked which caber he wanted to start with, piped up and said, "The biggest one ya got." Al wasn't willing to back down from the challenge and at least got the caber picked and attempted a toss, but only Capes

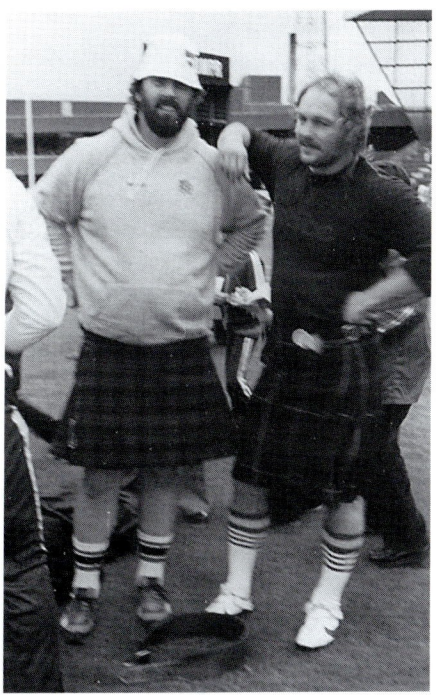

Al Feuerbach (r.) and Geoff Capes (l.).

was able to turn it that day. Al enjoyed the experience and would have done it again had the opportunity come up.

Today Al Feuerbach works as a freelance location sound recordist. "Location" means that he travels to the place where the event is happening. He has worked across the U.S. as well as in 60 countries around the world. He has been involved in some dangerous assignments along the way, including ones in Somalia, Bosnia, Republic of Georgia, Haiti, Chernobyl, Borneo, and Botswana. He worked with the news show *60 Minutes* in the 1990s on over 100 stories. Today, he focuses on sporting events. He has worked 13 of the last 14 Super Bowls for NFL Films, as well as numerous NFL games, major league baseball games, NASCAR, and much more. His job is quite physical as it involves handling a heavy boom pole that supports the microphone, carrying a mixer and wireless equipment, and moving with the action. Al said he most enjoys that his job is not only technically challenging, but physically taxing as well.

Al said he is excited about the current state of throwing and really excited about the U.S. shot putters, in particular Reese Hoffa, Christian Cantwell, and Adam Nelson (who is often compared to Al). Al commented that while distance is the most important, the classic glide has declined in form. He said you can't argue with distance and that's all that ultimately matters, but he misses the classic glide. Al has recently started going to some throwing seminars and sharing his wisdom.

I really enjoyed my visit with Al Feuerbach. I think the thing I enjoyed most was Al's approach to throwing. He didn't just try to copy what was perceived as good form but to expand on it, evolve it. Al Feuerbach was, indeed, an evolutionary thrower and he bridged that gap between the successful thrower and the successful weightlifter, a feat rarely accomplished so well. **M**

> AL FEUERBACH WAS, INDEED, AN EVOLUTIONARY THROWER AND HE BRIDGED THAT GAP BETWEEN THE SUCCESSFUL THROWER AND THE SUCCESSFUL WEIGHTLIFTER . . .

Dip, Grip, and Rip!

Pavel

What would happen if you replaced the gunpowder in a bullet with a high explosive? The gun would blow up in your hands.

Gunpowder is a propellant. It is designed to move an object instead of annihilate it. It burns slowly enough to be called a "low explosive," whereas a high explosive burns up in a fraction of the time of gunpowder, creating higher pressure and blowing things up.

These fireworks offer us useful analogies for two types of explosive deadlifts. A low-explosive deadlift is characterized by a controlled squeeze off the platform followed by maximal acceleration. A high explosive deadlift—"dip, grip, and rip"—is the subject of this article.

Why go ballistic

In the beginning of his powerlifting career, Mark Reifkind, *MILO* author and Master RKC instructor, had been accused by his fellow powerlifters of sneaking up on the bar and suddenly ripping it off the platform instead of squeezing it off. Rif laughed them off, saying that it was the only way he could ward off the "welder man"; he was not strong enough otherwise.

Belorussian powerlifting coach V. Dremach noted the same thing: a slow lift-off demanded great leg strength, and an athlete's back was often stronger than his legs. He conducted an experiment in which the athletes were instructed to perform the lift-off with a brief, explosive effort and then accelerate. The subjects' deadlift maxes quickly rose 15% and they now could perform several reps with their old 1-RMs! (Dremach, 1998).

No one can accuse Garry Frank of having weak legs, yet he also uses a lot of snap and jerk off the bottom as opposed to a squeeze. This dangerous type of start—called ballistic—obviously works for some. Let us agree with the definition by Belgian scientists Michaël Van Cutsem and Jacques Duchateau:

> RIF LAUGHED THEM OFF, SAYING THAT IT WAS THE ONLY WAY HE COULD WARD OFF THE "WELDER MAN"; HE WAS NOT STRONG ENOUGH OTHERWISE.

"A contraction performed as fast as possible, often called a ballistic contraction, is characterized by a brief contraction time and high rate of force development that is followed rapidly by complete muscle relaxation. Ballistic... discharge... takes advantage of a more efficient mechanical summation of the units' contractions." (Desmedt & Godaux, 1977)

So the upside of a snap and jerk start is a greater starting strength.

But it is over too soon

The downside, apart from the possibility of ripping something, is what neuroscientists call a ballistic contraction's short "decay time." Generally speaking, the more ballistic–explosive your start, the sooner your effort will peter out. You will have no grinding endurance to speak of.

To understand a ballistic contraction, it helps to know that the word *ballistic* came from the Greek word for throw. In a throw the force is applied briefly, and then the projectile flies on its own. If the projectile weighs 300 kg, good luck to its flying!

Belgian scientists John Desmedt and Emile Godaux discovered that while in a ramp contraction (geek speak for "smoothly increasing"), the active motor units increased their firing rate as the contraction went on; in a ballistic contraction the motor units started firing with great frequency, which dropped rapidly afterward. The muscles went from, "Hi! My name is Bob," to "Let's have three kids and a house in the suburbs," to "Nice knowing you" in the blink of an eye. You ripped that deadlift off the platform like it was nothing but ran out of juice before you got it to your knees. It is not just an issue of special endurance, but a neurological phenomenon programmed with intention.

There are a couple of ways of dealing with the decreased acceleration. One is perfecting the technique in such a way that the lift is performed in one gear—the initial explosion and the finish blur into one. This requires a movement where all muscle groups work seamlessly, rather than pass the load to each other in a relay. Tom Eiseman has such technique, as seen in a YouTube video (http://www.youtube.com/watch?v=8FjvxQpDmtM). "The lift . . . should be one movement," stresses the great deadlifter. "No shifting gears."

If you can't finish your high-explosive pull in one gear, former coach of the U.S. women's IPF team Mark Reifkind stresses that you must at least get the bar past your knees—and then you will have enough leverage to have a shot at grinding to the top successfully. Cheryl Anderson, pulling more than triple her bodyweight (320 lb. at 97 lb.), shows how to completely switch gears once the launch burst has died out and grind to the top with muscles other than the ones that have started the job, as seen on YouTube (http://rifsblog.blogspot.com/search?q=cheryl+anderson).

If the bar does not budge after half a second or so, you are going nowhere; your ballistic start will die on the platform. A ballistic intention, by definition, will not turn into a sustained effort. The welder man has won.

Pre-tension or not?

In the words of Tom Eiseman, who has been knocking on the 800-lb. door at 181 lb. bodyweight, "Your body should be semi-relaxed, as if you were ready for a burst of energy, like a sprint . . . contracting the muscles too much and at the wrong time interferes with your effort."

What is that all about? Don't we need to be tight?

> You ripped that deadlift off the platform like it was nothing but ran out of juice before you got it to your knees.

Here is the dilemma of the "dip, grip, and rip" puller. On the one hand, he cannot generate great force out of nothing: ". . . the absolute torque achieved during the ballistic contraction superimposed on the sustained contraction was ~25% greater than from a resting condition." (Van Cutsem & Duchateau, 2005) Prof. Verkhoshansky writes:

"It is known that a working effort must be preceded by certain changes in the muscle. They manifest themselves, among other things, in preliminary tension (anticipatory muscle tuning, according to N. A. Bernshtein) . . . if an active movement begins when the muscles are in a relaxed state, the latter are not ready for work and provide a smaller kinetic effect than they are capable of. It should be noted that the greater the resistance they overcome, the greater is the kinetic effect difference."

In other words, the heavier it gets, the more pre-tension matters.

On the other hand, there must be a brief relaxation of tension—a silent pause, as neuroscientists call it—an internal wind-up of sorts, before you hit it. If you are interested in the science, find the Van Cutsem & Duchateau (2005) study online and peruse their references. Otherwise, here are some analogies to drive the point home.

Watch a cat before he attacks. The predator is not rag-doll loose. Waves of tension and relaxation ripple through his muscles. He will briefly "press the clutch" for a split second to switch gears before the attack.

An experienced boxer keeps "dancing" his muscles, twitching them between tension and relaxation.

A seasoned wrestler will foresee his opponent's move once the former senses a sudden relaxation of grip and tension.

A good powerlifting example is a squat with a bounce out of the hole. If you go down loose from the start, you will get buried. If you go down tight and then smoothly reverse, you need to be one strong dude like Kirk Karwoski. If you go down tight, then loosen up an inch or two above parallel, you will drop and explosively rebound; you will get the best of both worlds—tension and explosion.

In plain English, pre-tension does not make you explosive and neither does relaxation; you need one before the other. It is interesting that not everybody exhibits a silent pause—it might be a learned skill rather than an automatic event. (Mortimer, et al. 1987; Walter, 1989; Moritani, 1993).

It stands to reason that if you have maximally pre-tensed, you will have a hard time releasing enough tension for the silent pause. I have experimented with ballistic deadlift starts from maximal preloading and they decidedly did not work. They worked more like grinds or low explosives. For humor's sake, I experimented with decidedly dangerous starts from a relaxed state. Predictably, not only was the explosion lame, but my spine bent like a noodle.

> WATCH A CAT BEFORE HE ATTACKS. . . . HE WILL BRIEFLY "PRESS THE CLUTCH" FOR A SPLIT SECOND TO SWITCH GEARS BEFORE THE ATTACK.

Professor Stuart McGill might have the answer regarding the pre-tension's sweet spot. He approaches the issue from an engineer's, rather than a neuroscientist's, point of view:

"Storage of elastic energy in a compliant spring, or a soft spring, is rapidly dissipated or lost. This happens if the muscle is not activated to a sufficient level. If the spring is too stiff, elastic energy storage is hampered because there is minimal elasticity and no movement (for the biomechanists, this is because the integral of the force–displacement curve is compromised). So, the pre-contraction level of the muscle just prior to the loading phase is extremely important. Another phenomenon is linked with this process. Interestingly enough, the pre-contraction level, and the resulting stiffness and stability, is a non-linear function that asymptotes. In other words, a lot of stiffness and stability is achieved in the first 25% of the maximum contraction level. From our work examining several different rapid-loading situations, it appears that a pre-contraction level of about 25% MVC [maximal voluntary contraction] creates the amount of muscle stiffness for optimal storage and recovery of elastic energy in the core muscles (at least in many situations). Less than this results in a spongy system, while more than this creates stiffness that impedes energy return and also unnecessarily crushes the spine and the joints."

A 25% pre-tension may be it and may not be. Dr. McGill adds that the above passage was "specifically for storage and recovery in the abdominal wall during things like throwing. I think powerlifting is different. You need the stiffness and pressurizing to a very high level to ensure the spine does not buckle . . ."

A personal experience

I had always been a grinder, but following a couple of years' layoff from pulling due to an elbow injury, I suddenly started "dipping, gripping, and ripping." It just felt right, since I did not have much meat in the glutes or quads. Marty Gallagher, who handled me at a couple of meets, pointed out to me that explosiveness appeared to be my trump card.

> THE TECHNIQUE WAS ADDICTIVE; IT'S A LOT MORE FUN TO FLY THROUGH A REP THAN TO STRAIN THROUGH IT.

The technique was addictive; it's a lot more fun to fly through a rep than to strain through it. Yet soon, at a point way below my old grinding max, the pull hit the wall. To date, I have wasted a couple of years trying to fine-tune the jerk-and-snap technique and the training for it. Not any more.

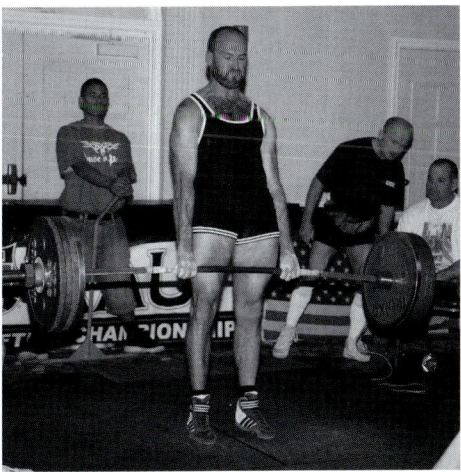

I dipped, I gripped, I ripped, and all I got was this lousy 501 lb. at 181 lb. raw.
Photo by CSS Photo Design, courtesy PowerbyPavel.com.

Perhaps it is for the leg pullers only

I am a back puller. Perhaps—only if your legs are strong enough to really throw the barbell off the platform—you can go truly ballistic and benefit from it.

Says Mark Philippi, "I think it is determined by body leverages, technique, and how many drugs you are willing to take—then you can lift any way you want and be successful . . . I think if you are a leg-dominant deadlifter, you may want to drive with the legs explosively, while back deadlifters tend to lock in, or using your terminology, wedge yourself in and pull under control."

Ukrainians Glyadya and Prof. Starov are on the same page:

". . . in the deadlift, the barbell must be accelerated to get through the sticking point . . . if the athlete pulls with his back, he needs to smoothly lift the barbell off the platform, increase the effort, and accelerate it in order to go through the sticking point with speed. But if the athlete pulls with the legs, he needs to powerfully rip the barbell off the platform (yank it off the platform), and then perform the movement steadily."

Not for everyone

It appears that a "dip, grip, and rip" deadlift is the domain of a very few talented athletes because of the conflict it presents. On the one hand, one needs to be tight to be stable; on the other, loose to go ballistic. If you are not succeeding in going ballistic, you are no longer getting the benefits of a greater firing rate and synchronization; so now being semi-loose no longer serves any purpose but to make you lose stability and leak strength all over the place. "I do not advocate grip-and-rip-style deadlifts mainly because the only person I have ever seen do it consistently was Dave Ricks," says armed forces champ Jack Reape. "Trust me when I say you all aren't Dave Ricks. Speed pulls aren't grip-and-rip unless you are special and freaky-strong like Dave, for which nobody whose name doesn't end in '-ov' or '-oan' qualifies." Watch Ricks pull on YouTube at http://www.youtube.com/watch?v=JVuI UdCIbaA&feature=related.

"Dip, grip, and rip" tips

If you insist on taking a chance, this should help.

- The high-explosive deadlift technique demands high excitation and does not tolerate complicated technique. The simpler, the better. Larry Pacifico teaches the triple-rock followed by a maximally explosive start. He told me it works for 90% of the athletes.

- A few subtleties: approach the bar breathing heavily, stomp your feet a couple of times, set your grip, wiggle your feet to wedge them against the platform, yank the bar a couple of times with your lats, then quickly raise your hips one or three times with an inhalation (if you pump

---

IT APPEARS THAT A "DIP, GRIP, AND RIP" DEADLIFT IS THE DOMAIN OF A VERY FEW TALENTED ATHLETES BECAUSE OF THE CONFLICT IT PRESENTS.

thrice, take in air with every pump and don't lose any), drop the hips, and hit it.

- The ballistic start makes it easy to let the hips shoot up and not use the legs and glutes. If this is a persistent problem, try the dive or modified-dive start instead of rocking. A static start is obviously out of the question.

- Keep your lower back flat!

- Switch to a double-overhand hook grip. Your biceps will thank you for it.

- Make sure that there is no slack in the elbows or shoulders in your starting position. Use your lats and triceps.

- Don't stay down longer than necessary. Not only would you be reducing the stretch reflex advantage, tiring and psyching yourself out, but also Prof. Verkhoshansky warns that "[the optimal preliminary tension's] duration must have a limit; exceeding it may significantly reduce the magnitude of the dynamic effort."

- As you hit it, think karate punch. The whole body suddenly turns into a solid block.

- Grunt or yell to start the lift. Not only has this has been proven to up your strength, you will get extra midsection tightness, which will make your spine happier.

- Use this imagery by IPF junior world champion Georgiy Funtikov: "Imagine that the barbell has frozen to the floor, that it weighs nothing,

> ". . . YOU JUST NEED TO BREAK OFF THE FROZEN-TO-THE-FLOOR BAR—WHAT CAN BE SIMPLER!"

you just need to break off the frozen-to-the-floor bar—what can be simpler!"

Ease into high-explosive pulling

V. Dremach advocates a slow squeeze-off start followed by acceleration for beginners and intermediates, up to Level 1. The coach insists that it is essential for proper technique development and safety. Then he switches his athletes to the explosive start and recommends special exercises for its development.

Larry Pacifico does the same. He has beginners do grinds—bodybuilding and core work—for three to six months to prep for explosive stuff. He then has them do plyometrics, and only after that does he introduce them to explosive pulls. But first he trains them to squeeze off and explode, and then evolve from it.

An alternative to "sneaking up on the bar"—get stronger

"Doing tons of box squats really helped my starting strength as well as my back and hip strength, allowing me to use a more reliable form," recalls Rif. He adds that once his squats and good mornings climbed, he had an easier time grinding his pulls and did not have to sneak up on the bar any more.

When everything else fails—just get stronger.

Jon Bruney

Foundations:
Speed, the Missing Piece of the Strength Training Puzzle

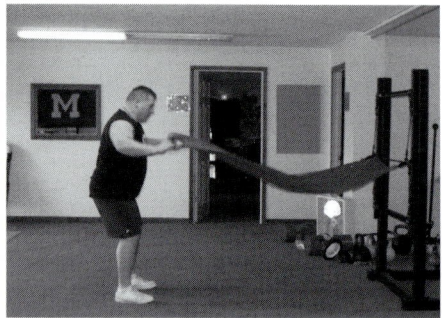
Upper-body velocity swiping.
Leona Sattison photos.

I believe that many strength athletes become one dimensional when it comes to performance. True strength training requires focusing on the lifts that require grinding strength, such as presses, squats, and deadlifts. However, grinding strength is only one piece of the training puzzle. To be a complete athlete you must also incorporate speed into your workouts. Speed lifts and exercises focus on building fast-twitch muscle fibers. These muscle fibers are often ignored in many strength programs. In this edition of "Foundations," I will be introducing some key exercises that will take your training to the next level. These exercises will build new muscle, burn fat, and raise your heart rate.

The first exercise is called upper-body velocity swiping. I was first introduced to the basic velocity-swiping exercise by Ori Hofmekler, who developed this exercise using a towel. I invented a special machine to take the exercise to a whole new level (see www.youtube.com/watch?v=iUCKPIAuyOQ). To begin, grab the handles of the canvas attached to the machine. Make waves by snapping your arms from chest level to waist level. The waves should be as fast as possible in rapid-fire motion. Keep making waves until you start to slow down. Repeat for as many sets as possible. This exercise sounds easy, but it is brutal. I brought the machine to a mixed martial arts event and created a contest to see who could go the longest. The best time was around 43 seconds. Most of the people who tried it were in good shape. This machine will get you breathing extremely hard. If you don't have a velocity machine, you can improvise this exercise with a large canvas, moving blanket, or beach towel attached to a power rack with a couple of daisy chains.

The second exercise is cable combination punches. Take a cable set and place the cables across your back. Grasping both handles, explosively punch forward for combinations of triple punches. Perform as many sets as possible.

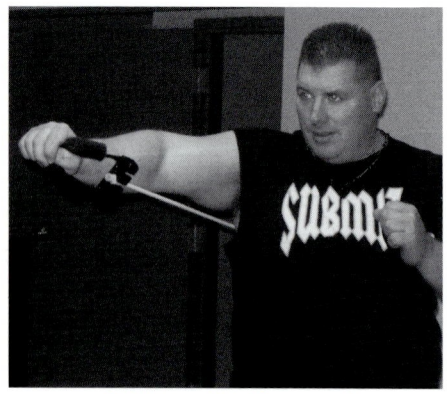
Cable combination punches.

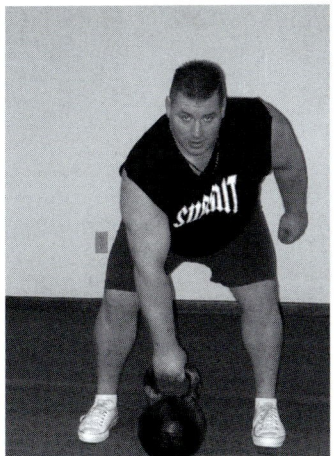
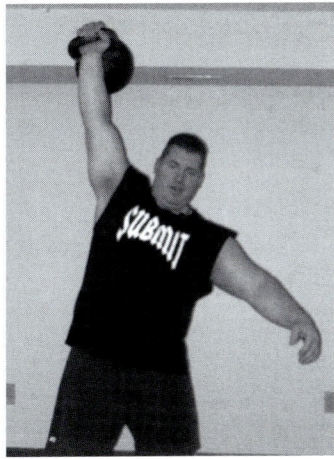

Kettlebell snatch from the floor.

The third exercise is the kettlebell snatch from the floor. Place a kettlebell on the floor just in front of your feet. Grasp the handle and rip it to an overhead lockout. Lower the kettlebell to the shoulder and then to the floor. Switch hands and repeat the movement. Continue to do the snatches until you notice your speed decreasing.

The fourth exercise is the sprint. Sprinting will build power in your legs and give you great conditioning. Perform as many sets of all-out sprints as your body can handle.

The last exercise is plyometric jumping. Squat down and explosively jump as high as you can while bringing your knees into your chest. As soon as you feel your feet touch the ground, explode up again. Do sets of 3 to 5 repetitions.

The best ways to incorporate these exercises into your training program are as follows:

- pick one speed exercise to do at the end of your normal routine
- make sure you go all out, do not hold anything back
- change speed exercises every workout
- substitute speed exercises in place of your normal cardio routine

Speed routine

upper-body velocity swiping	go for time until speed decreases, rest, repeat
cable combination punches	go for time until speed decreases, rest, repeat
alternating kettlebell snatches	go for time until speed decreases, rest, repeat
all-out sprinting	go for time until speed decreases, rest, repeat
plyometric jumping	3 sets of 5 reps

Organic Food and the Strength Athlete

Gabriel Josiah

If the words "organic" or "natural" evoke images of cosmetically-deprived women wearing tie-dye shirts and weird guys with hippie-length hair who burn incense candles, join the club—that's precisely what I thought, too. You, my friend, may have never even set foot in the singular world labeled the natural foods store, the land of bizarre citizens and strange cuisine. You might think the words "organic" and "strength" need never be paired in the same sentence. But, I hope to persuade you that going organic could be the smartest training decision you will ever make, even smarter than switching from leg extensions to 20-rep squats.

Take a jaunt to your neighborhood grocery store and you will see the organic and natural-food craze in fifth gear. Foods that used to just say "saltine crackers" now say "natural saltine crackers, made with 100% organic wheat flour" or "100% USDA certified organic ingredients." Next to the regular bananas, you see bunches of identical-looking organic bananas. But, unlike the low-sugar or the low-carb crazes, this trend is one you will definitely want to jump on and stay on permanently, even when it isn't in vogue anymore.

I call Auburn, Washington home. Auburn is a suburb of Seattle, the organic capital of the world. Okay, not really, but if you spend any length of time exploring Seattle's grocery stores, you will see that organic and natural are high on many shoppers' lists. I made my first excursion to a natural foods store as a youngster of nine. My mother (who, by the way, does wear make-up) dove head first into organic in the mid-1990s and let us tag along to observe this new world. After we got over gaping at the peculiar food—and the peculiar people eating the peculiar food—those trips actually became enjoyable.

I have something to confess . . . I have become one of them, those organically-minded people. Yes, I did grow out my hair (as Larry Norman says, "to make room for my brain"), but I just haven't developed an affinity for tie-dye yet. So, never being one to patty-cake around, let's jump right into this. What is organic?

> I HAVE SOMETHING TO CONFESS . . . I HAVE BECOME ONE OF THEM, THOSE ORGANICALLY-MINDED PEOPLE.

"If man made it, don't eat it."—
Jack LaLanne

You buy an apple—Red Delicious and non-organic, to be exact. Thinking to yourself, "This is an apple; man didn't make it; it's good for me," you sink your teeth deep into its crisp, juicy flesh. But did you know that contained in that solitary bite are chemical fertilizers (similar to the Scotts® you put on your lawn), chemical herbicides, insecticides, fungicides, and pesticides that are 10 to 100 times more powerful than the insect repellant Raid®? In addition, nearly all fruits and vegetables have been genetically modified to grow bigger and faster (bigger and faster is better, right?), totally against the natural course of things. Because of these factors, that Red Delicious apple has disease-causing chemicals and contains considerably less nutritional value than a Red Delicious from 60 years ago.

Let's examine just one class of chemicals used on that apple: pesticides. Pesticides, especially at elevated levels, are associated with cancer. The Environmental Protection Agency (EPA) has acknowledged sixty-four different pesticides as being "potentially carcinogenic," or cancer-causing. (1) More than 2 billion pounds of pesticides are dumped on our soils annually—that's roughly 7 pounds of first-class pesticidic goodness for every American. Maybe they could just give us a 7-pound tub that we could sprinkle on our cereal every morning. These chemicals are sprayed on crops to keep away—you guessed it—pests. But crop losses to insects and weeds have increased at a relentless rate, indicating that those darned pests are becoming more resistant to the chemicals (the insect rights activists love this). The response to these crop losses? More pesticides!

Of interest to milk lovers (doubtless most of us), a four-year European Union study demonstrated that organic milk contains as much as 80% more antioxidants (enzymes, such as vitamin E, that counteract the damaging effects of oxidation in the body) than traditionally-produced milk. (2) It has been said that you would need to eat up to five (!) times the amount of food your grandparents did just to receive the same nutritional value.

Let's look at meat. Just like the produce market, the meat industry wants to grow a lot of product cheaply, quickly, and with as high a profit margin as possible. That's reasonable. Unfortunately, this means using growth hormones to unnaturally accelerate the animals' growth; using massive doses of antibiotics to keep the animals healthy in unsanitary conditions; feeding the animals unnatural diets that pump more chemicals into the meat and upset the animals' systems so that they become unbalanced and diseased; and sometimes aging the meats, which allows deadly bacteria to grow. Virtually everything that you put in your pie hole that is not 100% organic has pesticides, herbicides, antibiotics, growth hormones, genetically-altered material, or chemical food additives in it—also known as toxins. All of these are the top contributors to sickness and disease.

Grab a box of non-organic cereal. Read the ingredients. If you cannot pronounce half the ingredients, it probably means they are chemicals. They are added to preserve the cereal and give it taste but they also suppress your immune system, making it more vulnerable to disease; they make you age faster; and they change your body from a natural alkaline pH state to an acid pH state, which means you are prone to cancer, heart disease, diabetes, allergies, and other sicknesses. (3) Many of the over-15,000 chemical additives used in foods aren't even listed on the label, a bit disconcerting if you ask me. Jordan Rubin, the celebrated author, includes a chapter in *The Maker's Diet* labeled, "How to Get Sick: A Modern Prescription for Illness." In it, he lists numerous ways to get sick. Guess what number 24 is? Eating non-organic food. (4)

Having said all that, 100%-organic food simply means this: food grown from the ground to your plate without the use of chemical herbicides, pesticides, insecticides, fungicides, chemical

> THEY ARE ADDED TO PRESERVE THE CEREAL AND GIVE IT TASTE BUT THEY ALSO SUPPRESS YOUR IMMUNE SYSTEM . . .

fertilizers, growth hormones, genetically-altered materials, or chemical food additives or preservatives—food that is 100% the way God intended it to be grown and eaten.

In 2005, my family and I switched to eating 80–90% organic foods. Thanks to this change (and the good Lord), we enjoy great health, are completely disease-free, and feel great! None of us takes any medication (not even Tylenol). None of us has had so much as the sniffles for the last four years. The last illness I had was a silly little cold that lasted all of one day. In the end, the results must speak for themselves. If something doesn't work, I want no part of it. When I eat non-organic foods for any length of time, I wake up the next day feeling dog-tired, sore-throated, and just plain crummy. It amazes me what a difference organic food makes. Not only is organic food better for your health, it flat out tastes better! Organic food tastes superior. It's like eating gourmet food all the time.

> WHEN I EAT NON-ORGANIC FOODS FOR ANY LENGTH OF TIME, I WAKE UP THE NEXT DAY FEELING DOG-TIRED, SORE-THROATED, AND JUST PLAIN CRUMMY.

Question: Is there a difference between being healthy and being physically fit? Answer: Yes, absolutely.

In the 1970s there was a well-known runner who could have run circles (more like miles) around most every man. He contributed articles to *Sports Illustrated* and wrote a book called *The Complete Book of Running*. He dropped dead of a heart attack in 1984. The man was obviously very fit, but regrettably, very unhealthy. Another instance of this occurred when recently a professional football player died of a heart attack while bench pressing. As strength athletes, it's all about adding the extra pounds to the bar, at times at the expense of our health. Let me clarify that I'm not referring to defective training methods, but to faulty diet: the quality of the foods we consume. Although eating organic may not solve the entire health puzzle, I believe it is the biggest piece of the equation.

> ALTHOUGH EATING ORGANIC MAY NOT SOLVE THE ENTIRE HEALTH PUZZLE, I BELIEVE IT IS THE BIGGEST PIECE OF THE EQUATION.

It's a given we all want to get stronger. But how can we improve, much less maintain our progress, if we are constantly battling colds, cases of flu, chronic fatigue, and other sicknesses? If you want to feel healthy, if you want to be free from sickness, if you want to eat fantastic-tasting food, if you want to be able to focus 100% on making progress in your training, and if you want to be fit and healthy, eat organic!

The mechanics of eating organic

Eating organic will cost more. Because organic food employs no chemicals, it doesn't grow as fast or last as long, thereby costing more to produce. But, hey, you either pay 15 cents extra for your organic apple now or pay much, much more in health care later on—

> COST WAS PERHAPS THE BIGGEST HURDLE FOR OUR FAMILY TO GET OVER. "ORGANIC MILK COSTS WHAT?!"

your choice. Cost was perhaps the biggest hurdle for our family to get over. "Organic milk costs what?!"

You probably will need to shop at a natural foods store for at least some of your food. Don't worry, the citizens of natural foods land don't bite unless bitten. Your basic grocery store will most likely carry organic fruits and veggies, organic milk, and some organic boxed or canned items, but you will probably need to buy all other foods at a natural foods store. Buy as much organic food as possible from a wholesale store (like Costco or Sam's Club) and you'll save a ton.

Reading the labels is very important, especially if you shop at traditional grocery stores. The food you are looking at should say "100% organic," "USDA organic," or "Quality Assurance International (QAI) certified organic" somewhere on it.

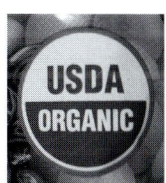
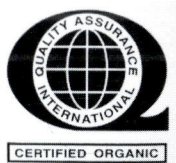
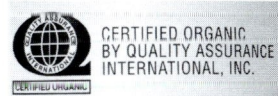

Organic-food labels to look for when shopping.
Courtesy of Gabriel Josiah.

More importantly, review the ingredients list. The majority of the ingredients should be listed as organic. There should be no words you cannot pronounce (which generally equates a chemical), no MSG (monosodium glutamate, also labeled as hydrolyzed vegetable protein), no aspartame, no high fructose corn syrup, no hydrogenated or partially hydrogenated oils, no natural or artificial flavors, no artificial color, and no enriched bleached wheat or white flour. If a product has one or more of these in the ingredients list, you should probably stay away from it.

This brings me to the question, "What is the difference between organic and natural?" As I said, "100% organic" means no chemical herbicides, pesticides, insecticides, fungicides, chemical fertilizers, growth hormones, genetically-altered materials, or chemical food additives or preservatives have been used in processing the food. "Natural" usually means just one of these processes has been used, such as no added growth hormones in milk or cheese, or no chemical preservatives in bread. But beware, "natural" can mean absolutely nothing. There is a procedure and standard for something to be certified as "organic," but for something to be labeled as "natural" requires no standard. I've seen "natural oatmeal cookies" that had a list of ingredients as long as Samson's hair, half of which were chemicals. Just because something is labeled as "natural," it doesn't mean that it's good. Optimally it should be labeled "100% organic" and have a minimum of ingredients. Organic and natural foods, as a rule, have considerably fewer ingredients than their non-organic counterparts.

> JUST BECAUSE SOMETHING IS LABELED AS "NATURAL," IT DOESN'T MEAN THAT IT'S GOOD.

Take a look at the comparison of two protein mixes below.

	Less than	2,400mg
Sodium		
Total Carbohydrate		300g
Dietary Fiber		25g

INGREDIENTS: Micro-Filtered Whey Protein Isolate.

Natural protein mix label.

INGREDIENTS: Metacarb-III™ (proprietary carbohydrate blend which contains: maltodextrin and modified food starches), PEPTOL-III™ (proprietary protein blend which contains: beef protein, whey protein concentrate, whey protein hydrolysate and egg albumen), whey, fructose, lowfat dutch cocoa, medium-chain triglycerides, natural and artificial flavoring, Metavite-III™ (proprietary vitamin-mineral blend containing: dicalcium phosphate, magnesium oxide, potassium citrate, ascorbic acid, vitamin E acetate, niacinamide, ferric orthophosphate, zinc oxide, calcium pantothenate, manganese sulfate, pyridoxine hydrochloride, copper gluconate, retinyl palmitate, riboflavin, thiamin mononitrate, chromium polynicotinate, folic acid, biotin, potassium iodide, cholecalciferol, cyanocobalamin), xanthan gum, cellulose gum, soy lecithin, salt, aspartame†, carrageenan, and acesulfame-potassium. Contains milk, egg, and soy derivatives. † Phenylketonurics: This product contains Phenylalanine.

Brand-name protein mix label.

The figure at the top shows a natural protein mix label from a natural foods store. The figure below it shows a brand-name protein mix from a supplement store. Whereas the natural protein has, well, protein, the other one has protein and about a hundred chemicals, preservatives, fillers, etc. (Readers beware . . . shameless plug follows. IronMind carries a high-quality, minimum-ingredient natural protein mix named, appropriately, Just Protein. I recommend it. And I didn't get paid to say this.)

You most likely won't be able to eat 100%-organic food all the time so don't go crazy trying; I don't want to read about your admittance into Bellevue. As I said earlier, my family and I eat approximately 80–90% organic. The other 10–20% accounts for eating out at restaurants, eating non-organic junk food occasionally, and eating whatever other non-organic foods might sneak their way in. Attempt to eat 80–90% organic; in other words, the majority of your fridge and cupboard should contain organic food. You could use the 10–20% balance for the foods that are prohibitively expensive in their organic form (organic protein mix, for instance). If for some reason you absolutely cannot buy an organic item, find a natural variety (no preservatives, no hormones, etc.). Yes, you will eat non-organic foods occasionally. Don't make a habit of it; otherwise, you are wasting your money on the organic food. Go all the way or don't go at all.

For the doubting Thomases out there who, like myself, aren't easily persuaded, read *Natural Cures "They" Don't Want You to Know About* by Kevin Trudeau and *Fast Food Nation* by Eric Schlosser. Also, watch the documentary *Supersize Me*. These materials are superb and can go into much more detail than is possible here.

In parting, seriously consider what I've said and look into it for yourself—you'll be pleased you did. Maybe I'll see you one day traversing the foreign land of the natural foods store with organic tofurkey, chocolate soymilk, and cod liver oil in your cart. If I do, no outbursts of affection, please—a simple handshake, slight bow from the waist, and "thank you" will suffice. And no jokes about my long hair and the whey protein-scented incense candles in my basket. **M**

Notes:
1. Don Colbert, M.D., *Walking In Divine Health* (Siloam Press, 1999), p. 106.
2. Eric R. Braverman, M.D., *Younger (Thinner) You Diet*, (Rodale, Inc., 2009), p. 110.
3. Kevin Trudeau, *Natural Cures "They" Don't Want You to Know About* (Alliance Publishing Group, Inc., 2004), p. 81.
4. Jordan S. Rubin, N.M.D., Ph.D., *The Maker's Diet*, (Siloam Press, 2004), p. 92.

> YOU MOST LIKELY WON'T BE ABLE TO EAT 100%-ORGANIC FOOD ALL THE TIME SO DON'T GO CRAZY TRYING

2009 Arnold Weightlifting

IronMind® Invitational: The Arnold Experience and Weightlifting Diplomacy

Matthias Steiner Meets California Governor Arnold Schwarzenegger

Randall J. Strossen, Ph.D.
Publisher & Editor-in-chief

Starting in 2003, IronMind has worked with Jim Lorimer to bring some of the world's top weightlifters to the Arnold for an exhibition on the main stage of the Expo Hall in the Greater Columbus Convention Center. That's a lot of words, but what it means is that Olympic gold medalists and the like are right there at the Arnold snatching and cleaning and jerking big weights with the sort of ease that only the best in the world can display.

In 2009, the spotlight would be on Matthias Steiner, the young man born in Austria who, moved to Germany for love of his wife, Susann, and his sport, weightlifting. Steiner had a dream he wanted to win an Olympic gold medal in weightlifting—but he felt that Austria was not providing the environment he needed to reach the zenith of his sport, so when he fell in love with a German woman, the pieces of the puzzle began to fall into place. Despite the tragic death of Susann in 2007, Matthias Steiner went on to win the super heavyweight gold medal at the 2008 Olympics . . . on the last attempt of the competition in what can only be described as a made-for-Hollywood story.

From there, Steiner's fame and fortune soared, earning him such honors as becoming the International Weightlifting Federation (IWF) Weightlifter of the Year, a *MILO* coverman, and Germany's

All photos by Randall J. Strossen.

Sportsman of the Year. His popularity swept Germany and he could go no place without being recognized and swarmed by fans and the media.

The prospect of having California Governor Arnold Schwarzenegger watch him lift at the Beijing Olympics had helped to fuel Steiner's final training as well as his gold-medal performance, but he still had not had a chance to meet his hero . . . that was about to change in a very big way.

Matthias Steiner, along with team leader Dr. Christian Baumgartner, coaches Frank Mantek and Michael Vater, media representative Marc Huster, and 2008 Olympians Juergen Spiess and Almir Velagic comprised the German delegation invited to the 2009 Arnold Sports Festival for the IronMind Invitational, the event IronMind has hosted on the main stage of the Expo Hall since 2005. As in past years, the weightlifting is the focal point, but these exhibitions are also cultural exchanges as much as they are demonstrations of the highest levels of athletic achievement. This year the German weightlifters dove into the Arnold weekend and the larger community with a packed program of training, goodwill, and camaraderie.

There was particular interest in this year's event because even though the IronMind Invitational had already brought six Olympic medalists in weightlifting to the Arnold, including three of the current men's gold medalists, it would be the first time we were presenting the sport's crown jewel, the reigning Olympic super heavyweight

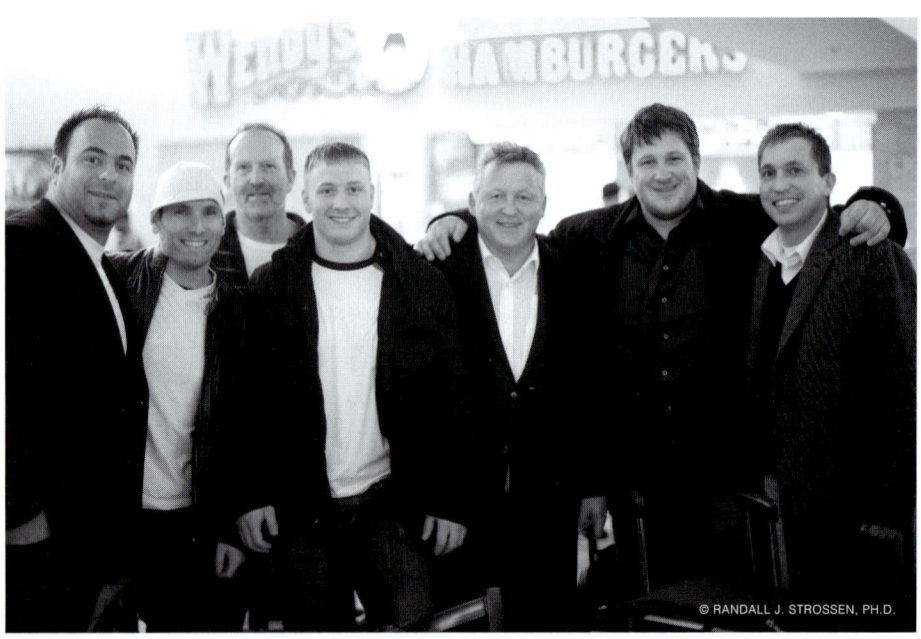

Just off the plane, our friends from the German Weightlifting Federation pose for the traditional IronMind Invitational welcome shot by Wendy's in the Port Columbus airport. Left to right: Almir Velagic, Marc Huster, Dr. Christian Baumgartner, Juergen Spiess, Frank Mantek, Matthias Steiner, Michael Vater.

champion . . . traditionally called "the strongest man in the world." Steiner's fame had already gotten him levels of mass media attention rarely seen in weightlifting. In addition, the German Weightlifting Federation represents, in IronMind's opinion, the most useful model for countries such as the USA to emulate if there is an interest in improving their fortune in the sport, so this was a unique opportunity for the sport's leaders in the USA to learn from the German Weightlifting Federation. Add to the mix Steiner's burning interest in meeting his hero, California Governor Arnold Schwarzenegger, and the stage was set for a standout production.

The German delegation arrived in Columbus, Ohio on Wednesday, March 4, and after getting checked in to the Hyatt Regency, we headed over to Barley's for its highly-regarded Kobe beef burgers and home-brewed beer . . . just the right meal for our guests after they stepped off their transatlantic flight.

The next morning, we walked over to the Downtown Columbus YMCA, where Executive Director Steve Gunn welcomed us. My friend Paul Travis had initially opened up the conversation for us with the YMCA about bringing the delegation over to train. Paul and I had trained together at the Whetstone Recreation Center (Worthington, Ohio) in the late 1960s (Paul was a very good weightlifter and I came there to squat and do an occasional power clean or deadlift); and he, along with his wife, Bev, were IronMind's point people in Columbus, offering everything from moral support to renting a cargo van if we needed to move our weights. Once again, the bond of lifting proved to transcend the limits of time and space.

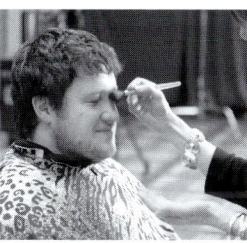

Matthias gets a touch-up before shooting a promo video for the 2010 Arnold Sports Festival.

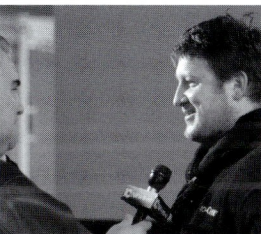

Channel 10 sent a TV crew to the Downtown Columbus YMCA to film the training session and interview Matthias Steiner for a story that ran on the news that night.

© RANDALL J. STROSSEN, PH.D.

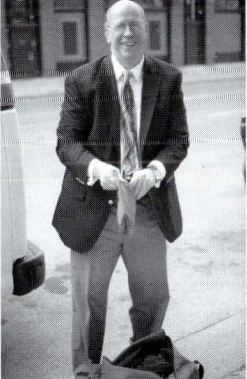

Paul Travis reached into his bag of tricks and pulled out his No. 2 Captains of Crush® Gripper . . .

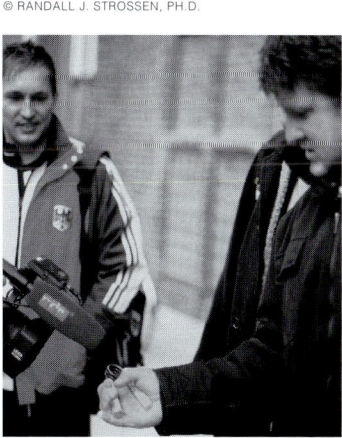

. . . which he wanted to see if Matthias Steiner could close. He could.

MILO | Jun. 2009, Vol. 17, No. 1   29

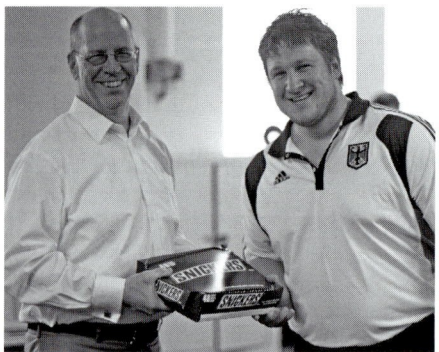

Matthias Steiner (r.), who is diabetic, was looking for something with sugar to eat, so look at what Paul Travis (l.) brought him.

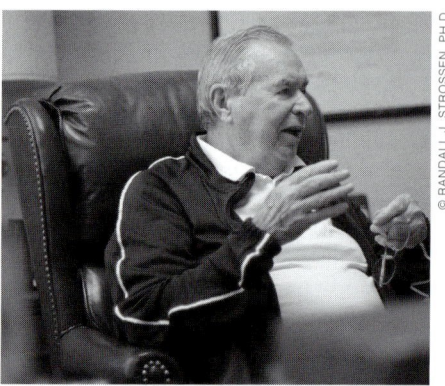

The man who makes the Arnold Sports Festival happen, Jim Lorimer invited us by his office as we headed from downtown Columbus to Upper Arlington.

Unbeknownst to me until shortly before his team visited the Arnold, Germany's head weightlifting coach Frank Mantek is a devotee of motivational psychologist Dr. Steven Reiss's work, and since Dr. Reiss is a professor emeritus at Ohio State University, Frank asked if it would be possible to meet the man whose work Frank considers pivotal to his coaching success. When I explained this to Dr. Reiss and said that we would like to invite him to lunch, he graciously accepted, so after the morning training session, we headed off to Upper Arlington and the Ohio State University Golf Club for lunch with Dr. Reiss and his wife, Maggie. Shortly before we left, we stopped by Classic Productions in Worthington so that I could introduce the German delegation to the man who made the entire Arnold Sports Festival possible: Jim Lorimer.

In the meantime, we received a very welcome phone call: the three competition sets that preeminent barbell manufacturer Eleiko of Sweden sent for the IronMind Invitational had—finally!—arrived. After getting delayed in customs and then taking an indirect route from the cargo liner to Philadelphia to Chicago and (backtracking) to

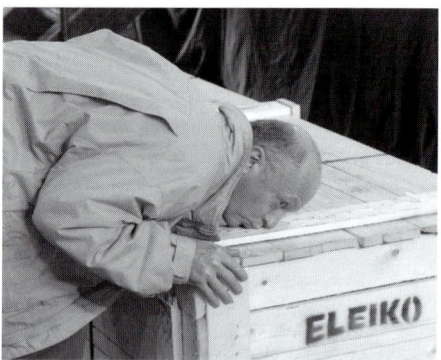

Eleiko makes the best barbells in the world and they kindly agreed to provide sets for the IronMind Invitational. Shipped directly from the factory in Sweden, they got hung up in customs until the eleventh hour, so when they finally showed up stageside, Randall Strossen gave them a heartfelt welcome.

Columbus, all surrounded by a blizzard of phone calls and e-mails—and thanks in particular to the persistence of one Deejay Adriano at our freight forwarder—the 1700-lb. crate was delivered with no time to spare on Thursday morning.

Thursday afternoon, we were back at the Downtown Columbus YMCA for another training session. Channel 10 was on hand for a story that aired that night.

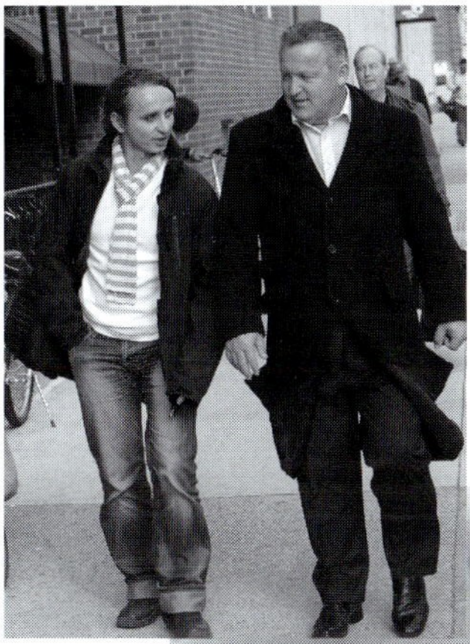

Ingo Hahne (l.), who headed up the German TV crew that came over to film the German Weightlifting Federation members at the Arnold, chats with Frank Mantek (r.) on the way to the Thursday afternoon workout at the YMCA.

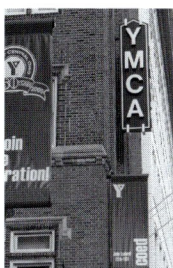

Back to the Downtown Columbus YMCA that afternoon . . .

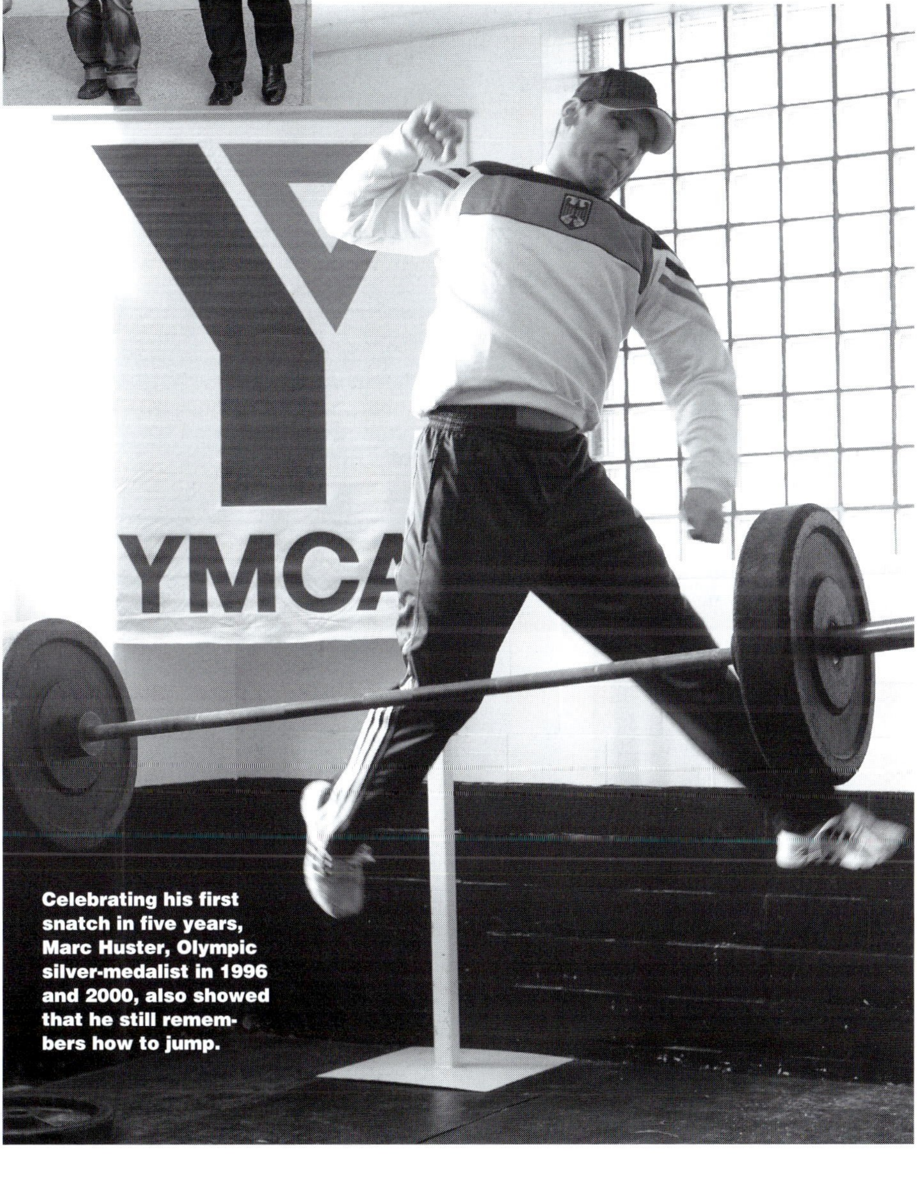

Celebrating his first snatch in five years, Marc Huster, Olympic silver-medalist in 1996 and 2000, also showed that he still remembers how to jump.

MILO | Jun. 2009, Vol. 17, No. 1   **31**

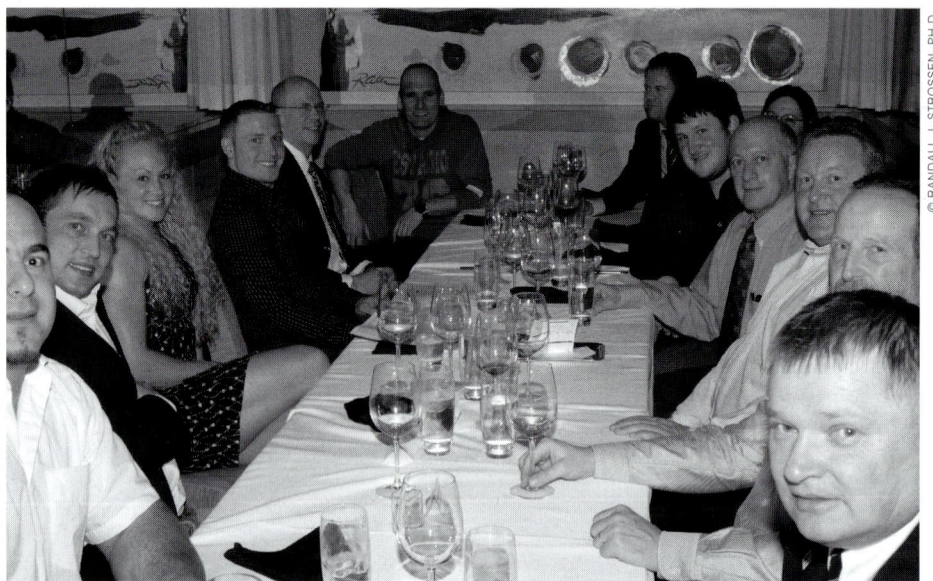

Dinner at M on Thursday: a private room, gourmet menu, and a lot of fun. Left side (front to back): Almir Velagic, Michael Vater, Ingrid Marcum, Juergen Spiess, Paul Travis, Marc Huster; right side (front to back): Dennis Snethen, Christian Baumgartner, Frank Mantek, Randall Strossen, Matthias Steiner, Bev Travis, Andreas Andren.

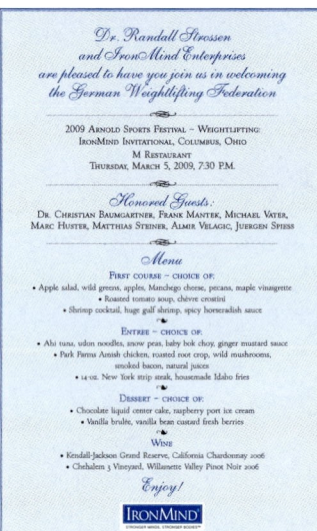

Thursday evening, our group and a few select guests had dinner in a private dining room at M, a Columbus restaurant we highly recommend for a special occasion.

On Friday the Arnold Sports Festival opened, so it was show time and after first meeting the Gillingham brothers at the GNC Grip Gauntlet, our whole contingent went to watch the preliminaries in the Arnold Arm Wrestling Championships, one of the sport's biggest and most prestigious contests. It is in fact the event that opens the Expo Hall each year.

At noon, we held a one-hour talk and question and answer session at the Strength Summit, which gave people a chance to ask these top weightlifters and top coaches whatever was on their minds. Many thanks to David Sandler and Strength Summit for taking us up on our offer and for making it all possible.

Participants had a chance to see the 2008 Olympics highlights video made of the German weightlifting team, and to learn, under Frank Mantek's leadership, how power and technique are

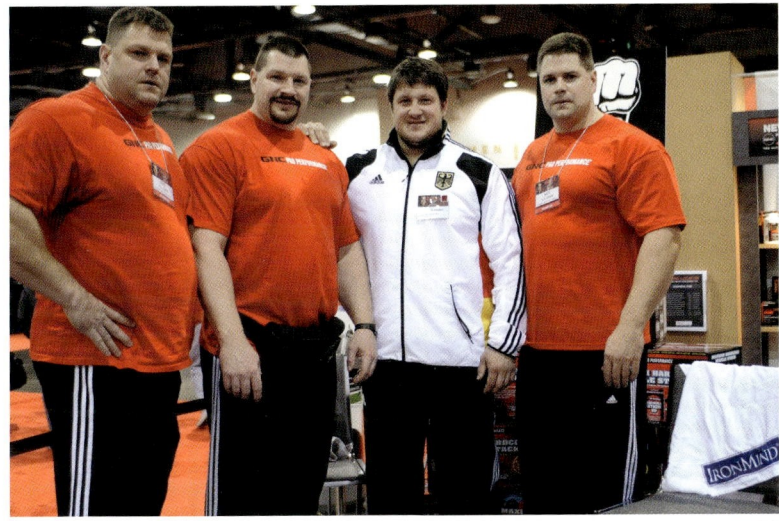

Our first stop was the GNC Grip Gauntlet to say hi to (left to right) Brad, Karl and Wade Gillingham. Matthias (second from right) looked at these guys and said, "I feel like a little kid!"

balanced in training; how the whole team works in unison; and how, possibly inspired by the German team's motto, U.S. President Barack Obama came up with a winning campaign slogan: "Yes we can."

Weightlifting in Germany is a meritocracy and if you don't perform at the expected standard, don't expect a free ride on the gravy train. While there definitely was a cultural-entertainment aspect to this trip, there was also a performance standard and the bar was set high. Head coach Frank Mantek wanted his lifters Juergen Spiess and Almir Velagic to lift under contest conditions and he had specific goals: Velagic was told that if he totaled 400 kg, he would be part of the German team going to the 2009 European Weightlifting Championships . . . if he didn't, he would be staying home.

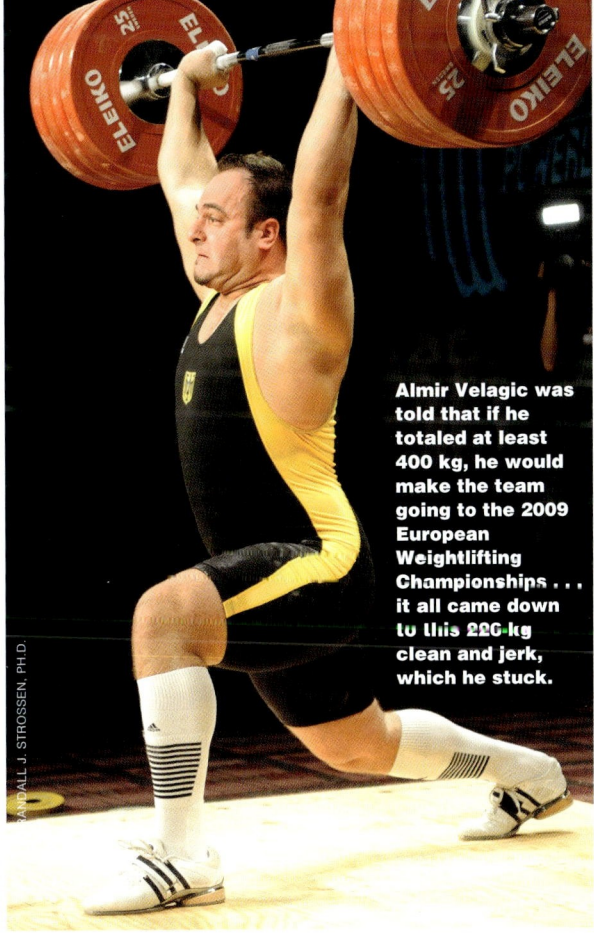

Almir Velagic was told that if he totaled at least 400 kg, he would make the team going to the 2009 European Weightlifting Championships . . . it all came down to this 226-kg clean and jerk, which he stuck.

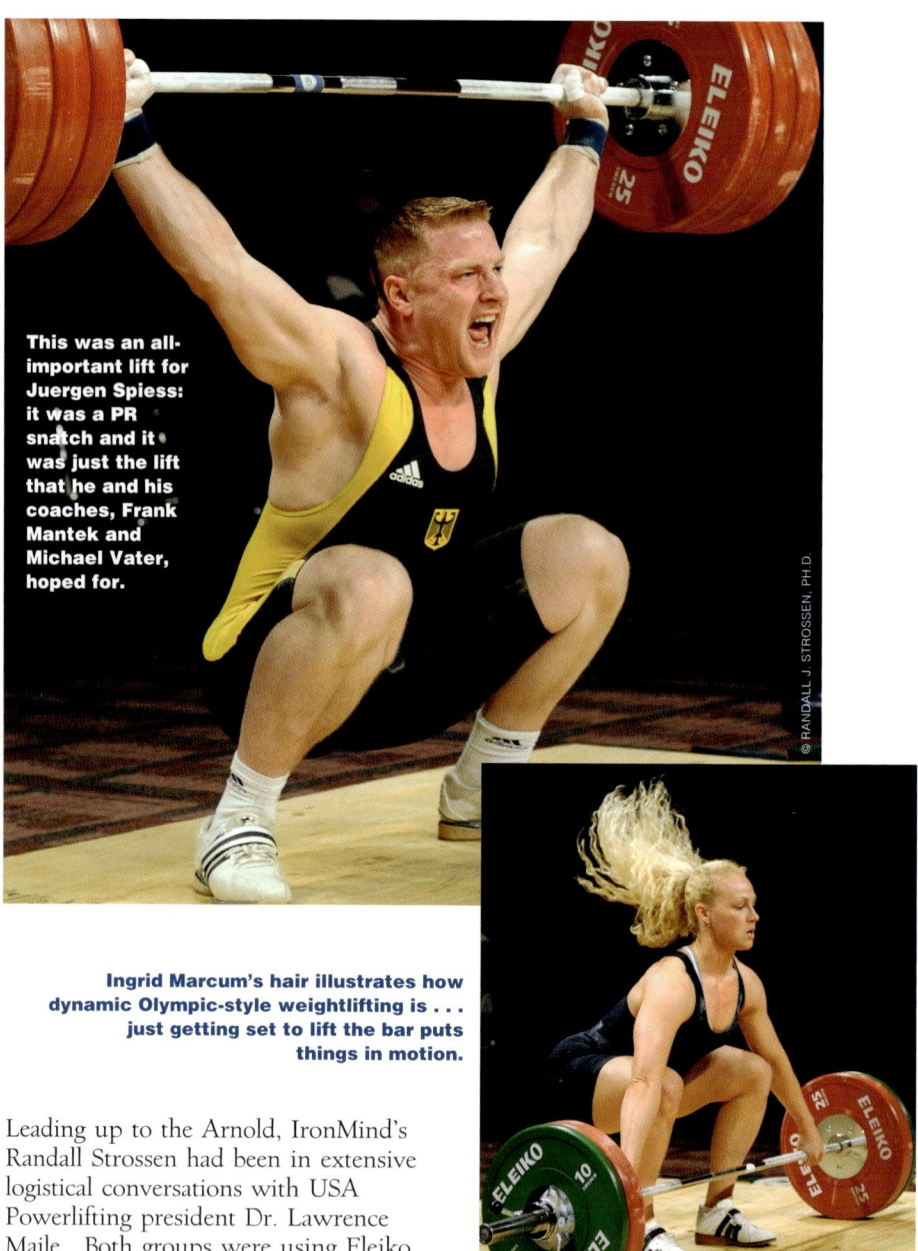

This was an all-important lift for Juergen Spiess: it was a PR snatch and it was just the lift that he and his coaches, Frank Mantek and Michael Vater, hoped for.

Ingrid Marcum's hair illustrates how dynamic Olympic-style weightlifting is . . . just getting set to lift the bar puts things in motion.

Leading up to the Arnold, IronMind's Randall Strossen had been in extensive logistical conversations with USA Powerlifting president Dr. Lawrence Maile. Both groups were using Eleiko barbells so to build on this common sponsorship and show IronMind's support for the USAPL (the drug-tested IPF affiliate), Strossen asked Dr. Maile if it would be possible for the German lifters to hold their control-level workout as a mini-contest in the Grand Ballroom right after the USAPL raw meet finished. Dr. Maile quickly and kindly agreed. Once over there, IronMind's friend Rick Fowler, who was announcing the USAPL meet, started waving the flag for us and before things had ended, thanks to Dr. Maile and Rick Fowler, new bridges had been built between weightlifting and powerlifting at the Arnold and beyond. In addition to its cooperative spirit, the USAPL is to be commended for its superior staging and lighting, the very elements we needed to elevate the feel and presentation of this competition to the next level. As serious as the lifting was, we also had fun: to keep thing humming along in between attempts, Marc Huster and I asked the audience weightlifting questions, with the winner each time getting a commemorative Matthias Steiner T-shirt or poster.

With our dramatic staging, a crowd that kept growing, and Marc Huster as the emcee, this was our dress rehearsal for the IronMind Invitational the next day, only the weights here were more than for real.

As part of the planning for the IronMind Invitational, Jim Lorimer had said we could plan on having California Governor Arnold Schwarzenegger meet Matthias Steiner. While security-related concerns would prevent us from knowing the details of when and where the meeting would take place, our hope was that it would be at the event itself. Saturday morning at 5:30 a.m. while cross-training by moving over 400 kg of weights by handcart from the powerlifting venue to the Expo Hall stage, I noticed that the bomb-sniffing dogs were already sweeping the area . . . a good sign, I

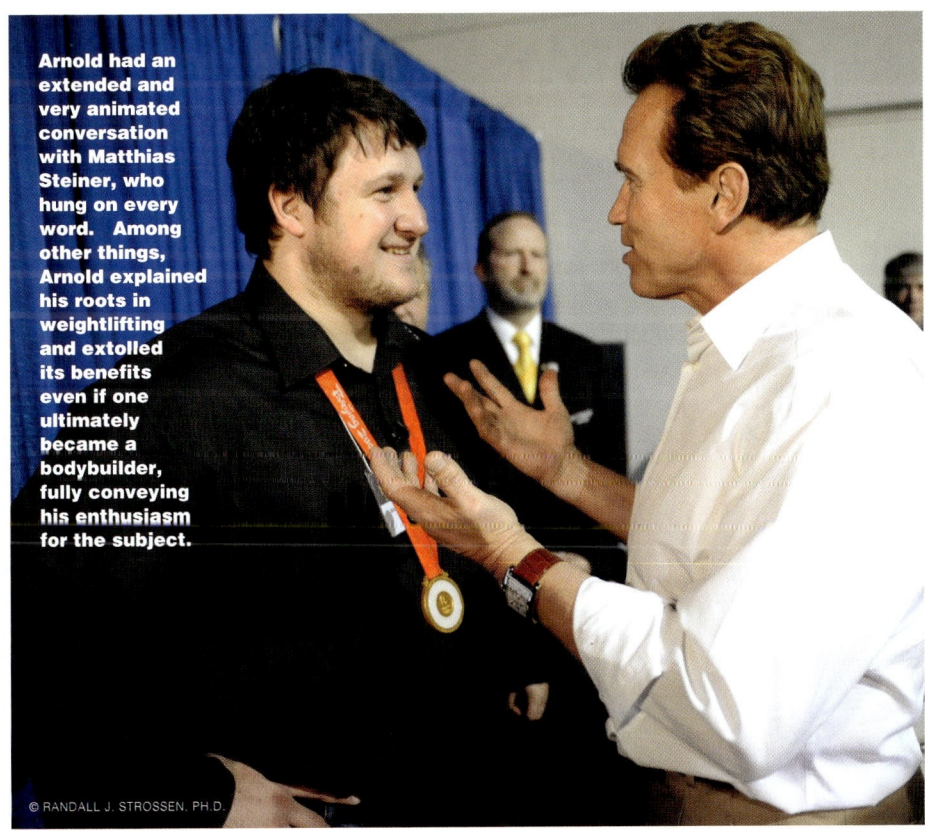

Arnold had an extended and very animated conversation with Matthias Steiner, who hung on every word. Among other things, Arnold explained his roots in weightlifting and extolled its benefits even if one ultimately became a bodybuilder, fully conveying his enthusiasm for the subject.

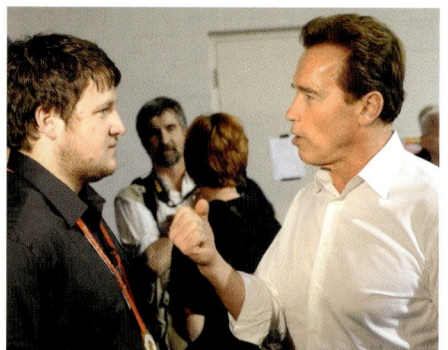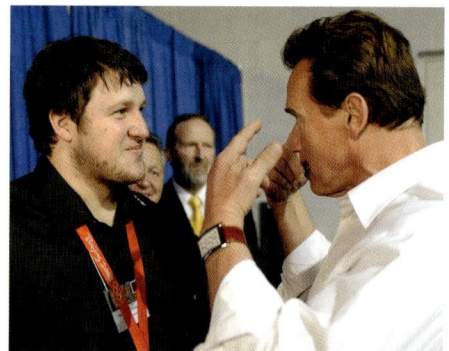

More conversation.

thought, and a few hours later, the scene and the reaction were repeated. I was starting to get a feeling that our wish was going to come true.

David Pursley M.D., besides being a neurologist, an IWF category 1 referee, and a licensed pilot, owns a plane, so when I invited him to referee for the IronMind Invitational, we got many talents in one person . . . and to give you an idea of his dedication to the sport, David flew in and out the same day just to help us. And if the weather had prevented him from making the flight, the good doctor told Randall Strossen that he was prepared to "saddle up" and drive the distance from Kentucky. Also meriting special thanks are Rege Becker and his crew of volunteers, strongman legend Brian Schoonveld for providing 350-lb. of muscle at our disposal, and strength coach Joey Soltis for showing the kind of can-do enthusiasm that is always welcome.

Minutes before we were to go on, Jim Lorimer told me, "Arnold will be coming down here, he will greet the Germans . . ." I quickly huddled the German delegation and explained what was going on; Almir stuck his fist in the middle and after touching up and going out with a cheer, we were off.

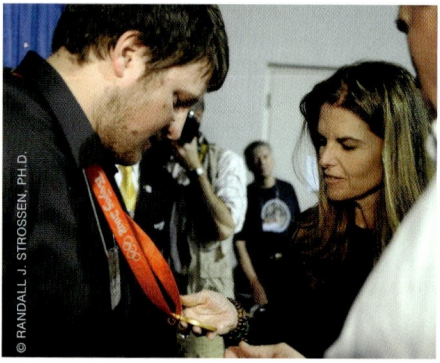

The magnetism of Matthias Steiner's Olympic gold medal was proven again as Arnold brought his wife, Maria Shriver, over to meet Matthias.

Arnold and his phalanx of security people swept in on the mighty wave that only Arnold can ride, and now Arnold and Matthias Steiner were face to face, speaking in Austrian. When asked later, Steiner said that at first there was a little lag time, but the California Governor was quickly up to full speed, fluently speaking his native Austrian with the weightlifting star. Arnold introduced his wife, Maria Shriver, to Steiner, and after minutes of conversation, the man who made his first name known worldwide took a ringside seat where he sat for the entire exhibition—a seal of approval that was not taken lightly.

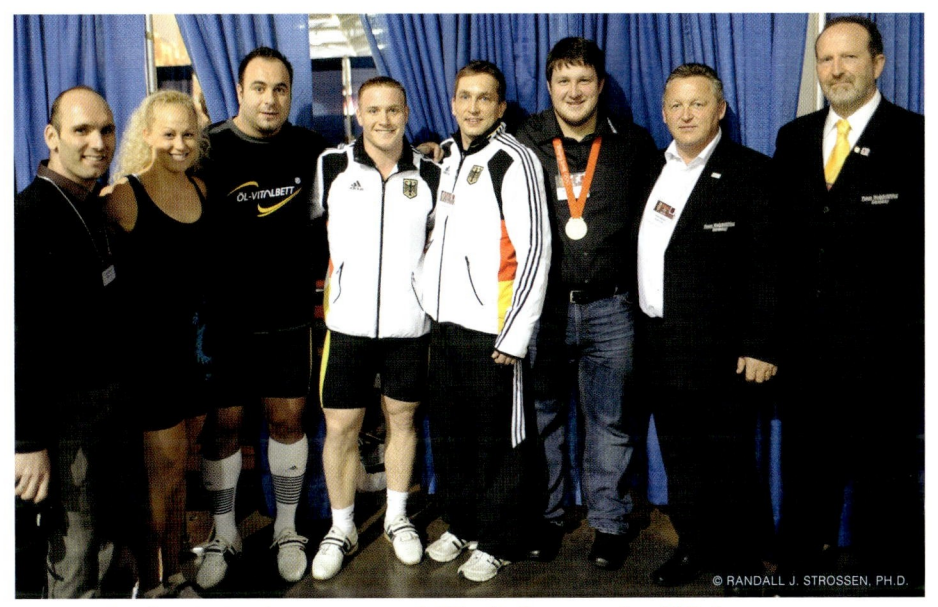

Having just had a chance to meet California Governor Arnold Schwarzenegger, our team was ready to roll on the main stage of the expo hall.

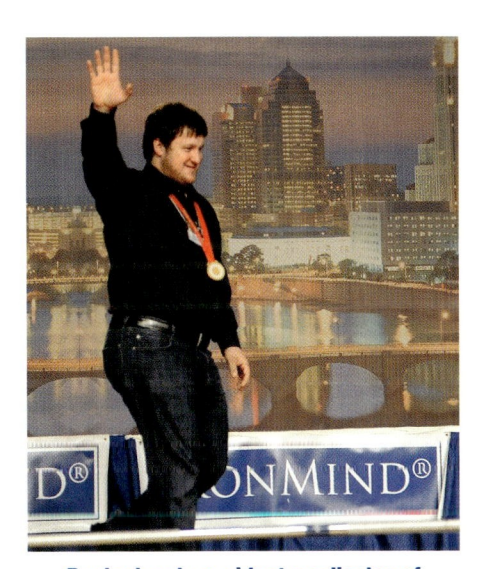

Backed up by a videotron display of Steiner's dramatic win in Beijing, the man himself was introduced to the crowd.

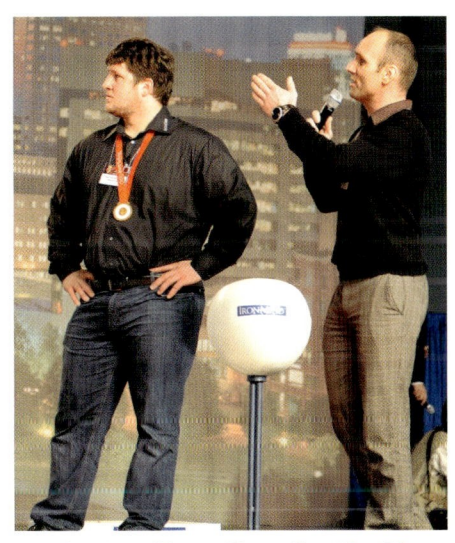

With Marc "Super Huster" putting his broadcast skills to good use, everyone at the Arnold got expert commentary from an Olympic medalist who also works as a Eurosport commentator.

The lifters: (left to right) Juergen Spiess (Germany), 2008 Olympian; Ingrid Marcum (USA), American Open champion and 2010 Olympic bobsled hopeful; Almir Velagic (Germany), 2008 Olympian.

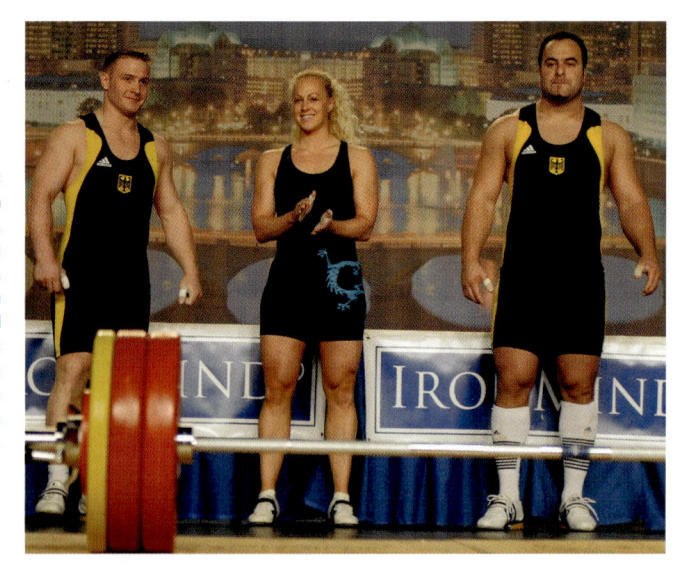

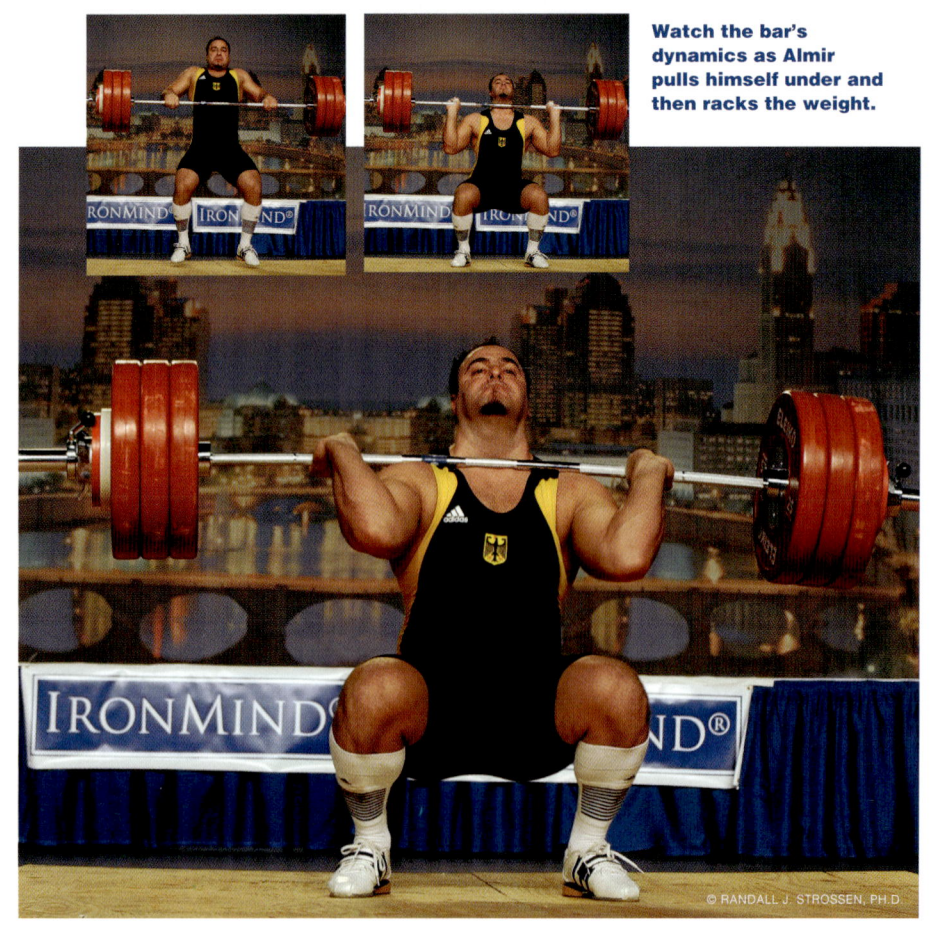

Watch the bar's dynamics as Almir pulls himself under and then racks the weight.

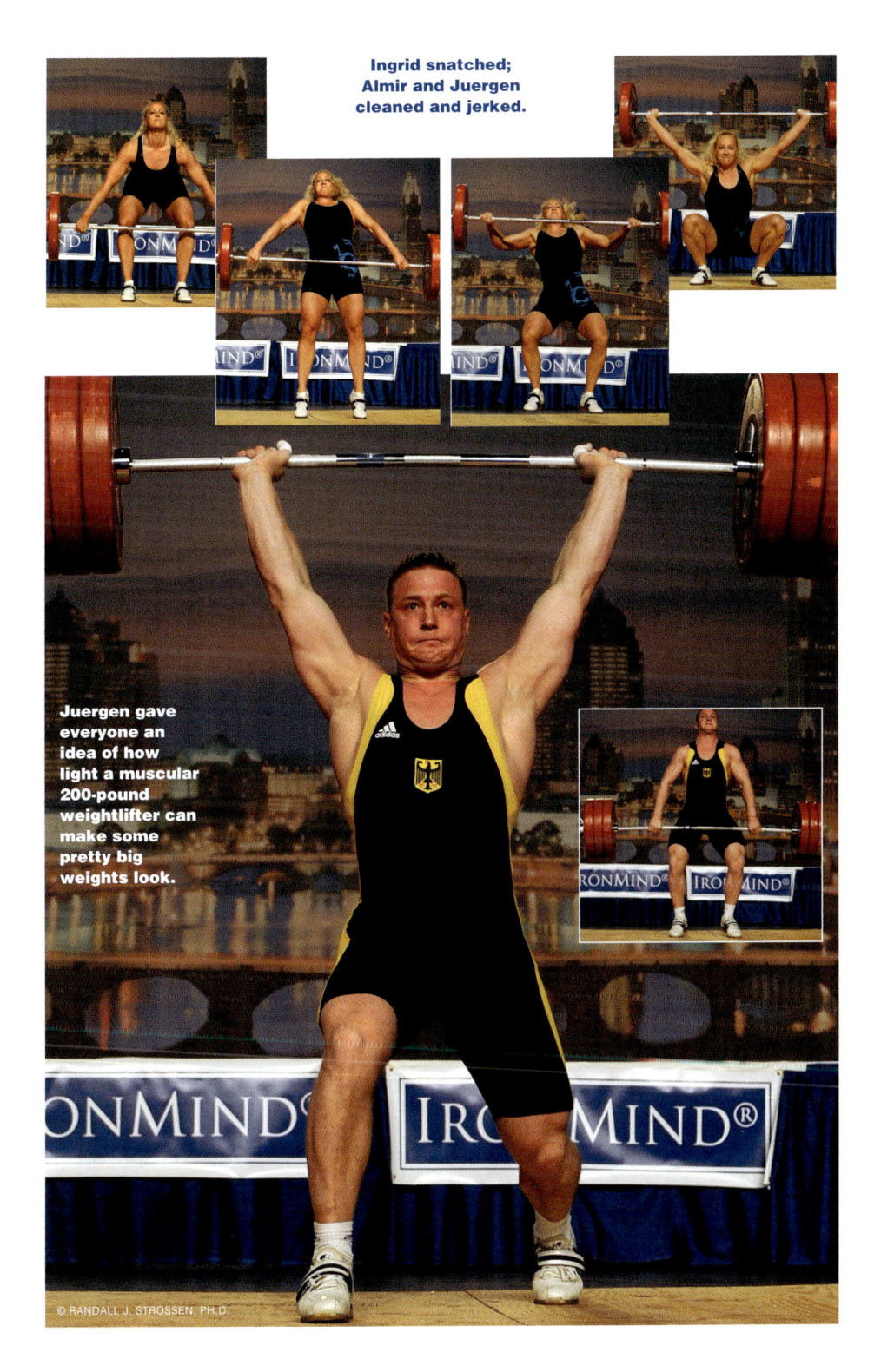

Ingrid snatched; Almir and Juergen cleaned and jerked.

Juergen gave everyone an idea of how light a muscular 200-pound weightlifter can make some pretty big weights look.

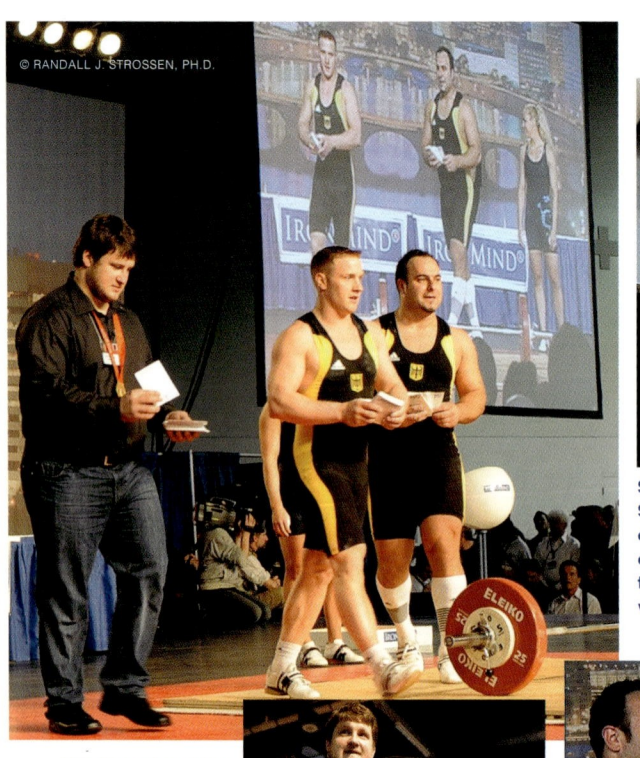

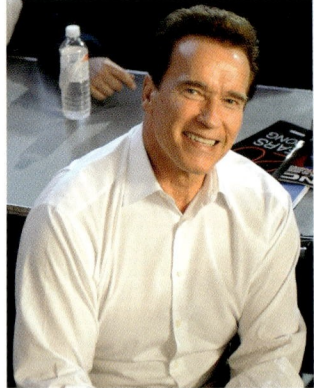

Sitting ringside, Governor Schwarzenegger watched the entire IronMind Invitational, once again showing his tremendous support for weightlifting.

It's the signature finale to the IronMind Invitational, something we've done since 2005 . . . the lifters feed the hungry fans with commemorative autograph cards.

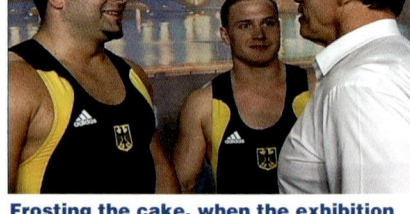

Frosting the cake, when the exhibition ended, Arnold came up on the stage and greeted each lifter.
Courtesy of Live! Technologies.

The exhibition was highly praised, not just because it featured the relatively low-profile but engaging sport of weightlifting, but also specifically for its cast: the two German Olympians and American weightlifter–bobsledder Ingrid Marcum, as all three showed the sort of wholesome athleticism that is every sport's and sponsor's dream.

By showcasing Matthias Steiner and his Olympic teammates at the 2009 Arnold Sports Festival, IronMind set out to create a very special meeting and an unforgettable experience for our guests from the German Weightlifting Federation, and to show how the sport could be used as a diplomatic tool. That's plenty, but we also wanted to demonstrate that this sport has a lot going for it—it can turn heads and hold one's attention. If nothing else, the IronMind Invitational at the 2009 Arnold Sports Festival proved that weightlifting is marketable well beyond its traditional limits. **M**

A Great New Way to Increase Your Bench

John Christy

In my now 34 years under the iron, I'll be the first to admit that very little is truly new. Even if something seems to be new, it was either done long ago or we simply hadn't heard of it. So when I say that what you'll learn in this piece is new, it is as such because I'd never heard of it or seen it recommended before (although some guy training in his garage in Cleveland or Budapest has probably done it).

The exercise I'm going to describe is one of the most difficult exercises I've ever performed. And as any experienced iron guy will attest to, when something is very difficult to do—and you master it—you can expect big strength and muscle gains in return.

The ironic thing is that I discovered this movement—what I'm confident will become one of the best movements you've ever hated to perform—out of necessity. What is the saying, necessity is the mother of invention?

Several months ago I injured my right arm and shoulder—a partial tear of the bicipital tendon—getting a dumbbell (DB) into position to perform an incline DB bench press. I've never been one to just sit around letting something heal while the rest of my bodily strength returned to my previous 118-lb. high school sophomore level. I devised a way to continue to train my entire body without any damaging stress to my right arm: hands-free front squats with a special apparatus; one-arm (left) pulldowns and T-bar rows; one-arm (left) shoulder presses; calf raises with a hip belt; back extensions; weighted sit-ups—and the unsupported one-arm DB bench press, to name a few.

I say "unsupported" because I couldn't use my right arm at all to stabilize and counterbalance the forces generated by using a heavy DB in my left hand. I couldn't hold onto the upright on the cage I bench in; I couldn't hold a DB in my right hand to counterbalance the weight in the left. Heck, the injury was so bad I couldn't lift my right hand to brush my teeth (seriously). I was forced to just hold it—carefully—on my stomach while I pressed with my left arm. The only other type of one-arm DB bench work I've ever seen is an alternating version: the trainee is still using two DBs and simply alternates pressing them—when one DB is at arm's length, the other is at the chest. In this version, both sides of the body are still balanced.

> HECK, THE INJURY WAS SO BAD I COULDN'T LIFT MY RIGHT HAND TO BRUSH MY TEETH (SERIOUSLY).

The alternating version is very different from the unsupported version because holding the resting DB in the non-working arm allows the trainee to counterbalance the weight in the working arm—and this makes it, well, easier. Again, as I described above, since I couldn't hold anything in my right hand to counterbalance the weight in my left, I just dug in my feet and flexed my core as hard as possible to stabilize myself, and went at it.

This movement was extremely awkward at first. It required that my pressing muscles and their supporting muscle groups work at a level I've never experienced before. And it also required intense, real core strength, because I had to fight to gain stability. I had to use the strength of my entire body to counterbalance the weight I was using in my left hand; my hips, torso, and lower body were trying to twist me into a pretzel. The only way to keep my body straight to avoid injury and to gain as much leverage as possible in the working arm (left) was to keep my body, and especially my core, flexed hard—very hard. And, boy, did I need to keep digging my feet into the floor.

I said this movement requires real core strength because I'm talking about strength built through the use of heavy weights on basic exercises, not through performing thousands of reps on all kinds of silly exercises. I'm talking about 150- to 200-lb. strict sit-ups; 120- to 160-lb. sidebends; 80- to 100-lb. back extensions (DBs held at the collarbone); and full-range arched-back good mornings using over 300 lb.—with all movements held in the contracted position for at least a full one-thousand-and-one count.

I want to make it very clear that I was not using this exercise to develop what is called functional core strength. I was using it to develop the strength of the pressing musculature that would carry over to the barbell bench (in my case, when my right arm was healthy enough to do so). I don't believe in purposefully distorting good exercises that are intended to work the torso, arms or legs just for a gain in functional core strength. I think that this has become a bad practice recommended by some respected strength coaches. My reasoning is that over-reliance on these fundamental movements (squats, ab work, DB bench pressing, hamstring work, all performed on a stability ball) will cause the prime movers of the torso, arms or legs to actually lose strength—for the supposed gain in this functional core strength.

The awkwardness created by having no leverage is what makes the unsupported one-arm DB movement great for building the barbell bench press, especially the bottom part of the bench press. As any trainee who understands the conjugate methods popularized by Louie Simmons's Westside Barbell Club knows, having no leverage is what makes some movements extremely productive in building strength that carries over to the barbell bench press.

As a matter of fact, the Westside program recommends a floor bench press to build the bottom of the bench press. The trainee lies on the floor with his legs straight out in front of him, thereby taking the legs out of the movement, which lessens the leverage generated by the legs when the trainee tries to drive the bar off the chest. I've utilized this movement— and it's good—but I feel the unsupported DB bench is better because you have less leverage not just from the legs, but from the entire upper body. And since

> And, boy, did I need to keep digging my feet into the floor.

> ... but I feel the unsupported DB bench is better because you have less leverage not just from the legs, but from the entire upper body.

DBs are used, the lack of leverage is most prevalent in the bottom position, when you are trying to drive the DB from a position that is at least a little below chest level.

The tremendous benefits

In order to maximize one's pressing ability, the scapula must be retracted (pulled together) and depressed (pulled downward), and held in this position throughout the lift. Doing this not only allows the trainee to maximize the strength of the pressing muscles, it also prevents injuries to the shoulder by stabilizing what is called the gleno-humeral joint. Squeezing the scapula requires great strength of the upper back musculature, and most importantly, it requires great skill that must be practiced to be mastered while using a heavy barbell. The unsupported one-arm DB bench takes this practice to a new level. The upper-back musculature will have to learn to flex even harder than required with a barbell in order to stabilize the weight's being held in only one hand. Without maintaining retraction and depression, to the point of cramping the traps and lats, the trainee has no chance of getting the DB with any appreciable weight out of the bottom position.

This movement will also teach you (should I say force you, again?) to learn what I consider to be the ideal 45-degree angle of the upper arm (humerus) relative to the side of your torso. Some benchers keep the humerus at a much greater angle—some nearly 90 degrees—because they feel that they can use their pecs better in this position. Experience has taught me that this is not optimal because you can't retract and depress the scapula maximally with the humerus at this angle. Also as the angle increases, huge and unnecessary harmful forces impinge on many structures in the shoulder, especially at the pec tie-off and in the bicipital tendon. When trying to stabilize one arm, you have to optimally retract and depress the scapula, and doing so will pull that arm closer (relative to a 90-degree angle) to the side.

> ALSO AS THE ANGLE INCREASES, HUGE AND UNNECESSARY HARMFUL FORCES IMPINGE ON MANY STRUCTURES IN THE SHOULDER . . .

If you're a bencher who doesn't use the triceps to their maximum, meaning that you don't focus on flexing or creating tension in the triceps when driving the barbell out of the bottom position, this movement will teach you to do that. As a matter of fact, it will force you to learn to use your triceps.

How to perform the movement

I would suggest that you use Powerhooks (from Country Power, Inc.) so that you can un-rack the DB in the top position. This way, you not only avoid having to put the DB on your leg and kick it up into position (although this is what I did for years—until this last injury), you'll be able to set up your body and retract and depress the scapula much more efficiently.

It really doesn't matter what you do with the non-working arm: just *don't* hold onto anything, including the pad on the bench. I had to rest mine on my stomach simply because it caused pain to put it anywhere else.

Before you begin the descent, squeeze those shoulder blades together as if you are trying to cause a spasm in your

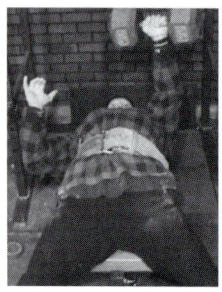

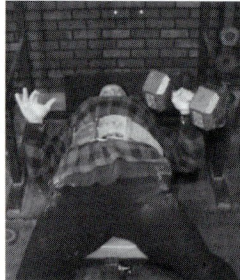

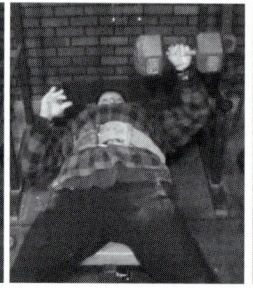

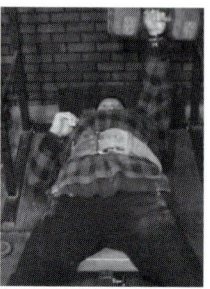

Unsupported one-arm DB bench, start to finish.
Photos courtesy of John Christy.

upper-back muscles. It'll be very hard at first to maximally contract the upper-back muscles on the side that is not holding a DB, but stay with it; you'll learn to do it.

As you lower the weight, you'll not only have to keep your entire upper back tight and your pressing muscles (the prime movers) on the working side tight (generating great tension, the key to great strength), you'll also be forced to keep your entire body tight, especially all the muscles in your core. And boy, will you have to use your legs and dig in your feet like never before! Your body will try to twist toward the working side as the DB reaches the lower position. Don't let it! Stand your ground and keep your shoulders and hips parallel with the ceiling. This takes tremendous concentration and, of course, tremendous core and whole-body strength. You'll find out very quickly how strong your middle is.

Now, to have any chance of getting a heavy weight out of the bottom position, you'll need to keep that upper back of yours in a near spasm. If your scapula pulls out even a little, you're done—you won't make the lift. The unsupported one-arm DB bench is very unforgiving; any flaws in technique or bodily tension and you will fail to make the lift.

Learning to maintain maximum levels of tension in the muscles that stabilize the parts of the body that allow the prime movers to generate maximum strength is what makes this exercise so productive for building the barbell bench press. Your upper-back musculature and the muscles of your midsection (your core) will think they are on vacation when you go back to pressing a barbell that has both of your hands/arms connected (both hands holding the same bar) and the weight counterbalanced perfectly between both sides of your upper body.

> YOU'LL FIND OUT VERY QUICKLY HOW STRONG YOUR MIDDLE IS.

How to fit it into your program

Incorporating the unsupported one-arm DB bench into your workouts is not very complicated. Use it as your stand-alone bench work for three to four months. Perform a set or two of 3 reps with 80% of your one-rep maximum (1-RM) once a week with the barbell as a warm-up for the DB work if you are a powerlifter or if you simply want to stay in the groove with the barbell.

> WHEN YOU GO BACK TO THE BARBELL (AS LONG AS YOU'VE BEEN DOING SOME PRACTICE TO STAY IN THE GROOVE), SAY HELLO TO A NEW PR.

If you follow any of the variations of the conjugate method popularized by Westside Barbell, the unsupported one-arm DB bench makes a fantastic maximal effort (ME) movement. I strongly suggest several weeks of using it as an auxiliary movement following your usual ME movement for several sets of 5 to 8 reps so you can develop the unique whole-body motor skills and strength necessary to make this movement not only productive—but also safe. You want to keep yourself from getting hurt, so please take the getting hurt part very seriously. If you rush into this with big weights too fast, or if your core isn't strong enough, you can kiss your lower back goodbye.

Once you get the movement down (and get your core strong enough), plug it right in as an ME movement. Simply work up to using sets of 3 reps until you can no longer make the 3 reps, and then perform singles until you arrive at your 1-RM. A great way to utilize this as an ME movement is to cycle it through a 7-week mesocycle using different angles of incline. For instance, you can start with a regular supine (flat) bench. Establish your 1-RM and then the next week use a 30-degree incline. The following week go up to a 45-degree incline. The next week push it to roughly 60 degrees, and then over the next three weeks, work your way back down, breaking your 1-RMs along the way. When you go back to the barbell (as long as you've been doing some practice to stay in the groove), say hello to a new PR.

The wrap-up

The DB bench press has been a staple in the arsenal of bench pressers for a long time simply because it is harder than the barbell version. Each arm, each side of the body, has to act independently to a degree to control each DB since there is no bar connecting each hand—and each side of the body. This requirement makes both the prime movers and the stabilizers work much harder.

The unsupported one-arm DB bench press is not just a step above its brother, in my opinion: it's an entire staircase above it. Again, when something gets harder to do, it will be more productive. The key is to learn to do it right, and then give your body time to adapt to the unique stresses placed upon it so that you can develop the motor skills and special strengths that are required to maximize the movement's potential benefits.

If you want to give your barbell bench press a big boost, try something new; try something that is very hard to do: the unsupported one-arm DB bench press. You won't be disappointed. **M**

> IF YOU RUSH INTO THIS WITH BIG WEIGHTS TOO FAST, OR IF YOUR CORE ISN'T STRONG ENOUGH, YOU CAN KISS YOUR LOWER BACK GOODBYE.

Pulling Sleds Made Easy

Ernest Roy, PT, DPT

One training technique highly valued for its ability to improve speed and acceleration power is sled pulling. A March 2009 *MILO* article by Matt Shatzkin ["Playing Around with the Push Sled," Vol. 16, No. 4] spoke of uses for pushing sleds like those commonly seen in football camps. For boosting one's quickness and bursting speed, however, sled pulls can make a great difference. What running back wouldn't like to be able to pop through the holes in the defensive line more quickly? Strongman competitors will appreciate that explosiveness in the medley events, where drag-and-carry combos require strength, quickness, and speed-endurance.

While helping my 15-year-old son put together a speed training program for baseball, I came across a small online article that talked about using an old tire as a makeshift pulling sled. With that spark of inspiration, we modified the approach, and I would like to share what we did with *MILO* readers.

The sled we devised has the advantages of being simple to craft, with only a few basic tools needed. The materials should be readily available and easy to find—we got them from our basement, local hardware store, and town recycling center. It was also very inexpensive, and in these times we can all appreciate that. The weight load is easily adjusted, making it useful for a variety of athletes.

> FOR BOOSTING ONE'S QUICKNESS AND BURSTING SPEED, HOWEVER, SLED PULLS CAN MAKE A GREAT DIFFERENCE.

The biggest component of the pulling sled is an old tire, which was given to me by the town recycling center. When I asked the fellow working there if there were any old tires he could let me have, he laughed and said, "Take your pick, there must be a hundreds of 'em out back waiting for the disposal truck." I offered to pay him for it, but he refused (it's always good manners to at least offer—never just raid these places expecting to walk out with whatever you want). To the tire we attached an old tractor chain (weighing about 18 lb.) that I got from my late father-in-law. The chain had a hook on one end, making it convenient to loop around the tire in such a way as to keep it from sliding off when dragged. The total weight of the tire and chain was around 27 lb.; this was perfect, since the training program we used called for a sled weight of around 15–20% of the bodyweight of the person pulling it.

As shown in the photo, I drilled a hole in one end of the tire and attached a screw-in hook, with a nut and washer on either side of the hook hold it snugly to the tire.

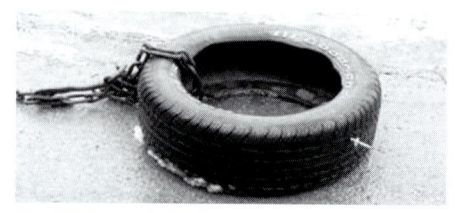

Basic tire and chain set-up: note the small hook screwed into the tire.

The next photo shows how the tire sled is attached to the athlete.

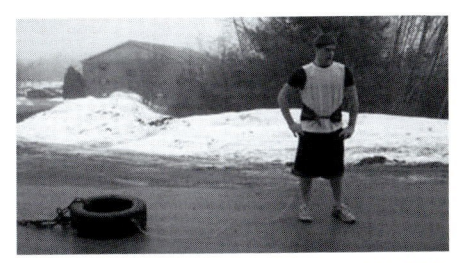

Tire attached to athlete's SUPER SQUATS Hip Belt and ready for action.

An 8' section of thin steel cable from our local hardware store was looped at each end and a screw-down clamp was attached to the ends to secure the loops. A clip was used to attach one looped end of the cable to the tire hook; the other looped end is clipped to the athlete's belt. We use IronMind's SUPER SQUATS Hip Belt for our sled pulls: it fits comfortably, adjusts easily and is as tough as a three-dollar steak. Whatever you use for a belt, make sure you get one that won't slip or break under the stress. You don't want to blast off the start line and fall face first to the pavement because your belt broke and threw you off stride.

The final photo shows Matt as he is coming off the line with the tire in tow. He's showing good starting posture: torso leaning forward, head relaxed, and arms pumping hard with each step. At about 10 m out, he will come upright as he gets closer to full speed and he will maintain this posture through the finish line (about 30 m for our purposes).

If you're curious about the program we're using, it's based on a well-written research study that looked at the use of various forms of resisted sprinting for improving top-end and accelerating speed (1). Two to three times per week, warm up and then do four to five sled pulls with a total sled weight of 15–20% bodyweight. Go as hard as you can for 25 to 30 m if your goal is to increase quick-burst accelerating speed. Rest 3 to 4 minutes between each effort —you'll need to if you want to get the most from each run. Try this for a six- to eight-week training cycle.

For those who want to focus more on pure strength, you could simply add more chain to the tire, use a larger tire, or try a combination of the two. One point that must be stressed for people whose sport demands high speeds (e.g., track, football, rugby) is do not use too heavy a load. Loads of over 20% bodyweight may alter your running style so much that it bears little resemblance to what you really want to do on the field. I should mention that, apart from the IronMind SUPER SQUATS Hip Belt, this set-up costs about ten dollars for the materials. Try this pulling sled if you want a low-cost way to add some variety to your training that will really pay off with some nice results. **M**

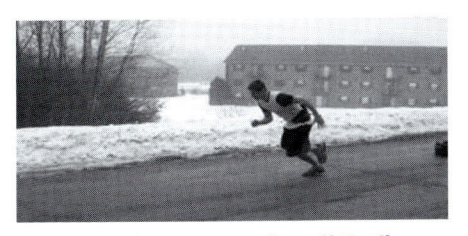

Use good posture coming off the line.

1. R. G. Lockie, A. S. Murphy, and C. D. Sparks, "Effects of resisted sled training on sprint kinematics in field sport athletes," *Journal of Strength & Conditioning Research* 17 (2003): 760–767.

Russian Men of Might: General-Lieutenant V. G. Kostenetsky

Joseph Svub

One of Napoleon's greatest victories occurred at Slavkov, a town about six miles southeast of Brno, the Moravian capital, which is a part of the modern Czech Republic. The battle of the Three Emperors, or as it was alternatively named, the battle of Austerlitz, occurred in 1805.

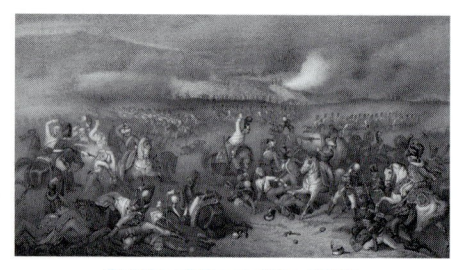

Battle of Austerlitz, 1805. It is in this setting that the legendary tales of Vasily Kostenetsky begin.

On December 2 of that year, a French army decisively destroyed a Russian–Austrian army commanded by Tsar Alexander I. Bonaparte initially met the combined Allied army of 85,000 men and 278 guns with just 66,000 men. Around 8:00 A.M., the first Allied columns began hitting the French near the village of Telnitz (Telnice) and threw the French back across the Goldbach stream. Around 8:45 A.M., Napoleon ordered an attack on the Russian lines atop Pratzen Heights. Then the Emperor remarked, "One sharp blow and the war is over," and ordered the assault to move forward. A French division managed to capture the heights. To the north, General Dominique Vandamme's division defeated the Allied forces around Stare Vinohrady vineyard.

The Russian squad commandant Colonel Vasily Kostenetsky, brandishing his unsheathed sabre, shouted in a terrible voice, "Storm!" The fireworker Maslov, reportedly a giant of a man similar to Kostenetsky, helped the horses pull the Russian guns through the vineyards. When the horses stalled, Kostenetsky assisted in moving the guns. While crossing a deep stream, Kostenetsky noticed that four guns were left in French hands. "Four guns to the delight of the enemies?" cried the Colonel. "Never! Maslov, forward!—I mean backward, to save our guns!" Thus two lone Russian soldiers, Kostenetsky and Maslov, ran back to their former positions, now occupied by Napoleon's troops. Many historians wrote with astonishment and misgiving, that Kostenetsky—who in the course of the fight lost his saber—took a huge wooden ramrod and began to smash enemies from left to right,

> KOSTENETSKY—WHO IN THE COURSE OF THE FIGHT LOST HIS SABER—TOOK A HUGE WOODEN RAMROD AND BEGAN TO SMASH ENEMIES FROM LEFT TO RIGHT, . . .

walking over dead bodies like an unstoppable colossus. French losses at the battle amounted to 8,000, while the Russian and Austrian emperors, present at the battle, saw more than 27,000 of their men killed, wounded and captured. Napoleon also captured 180 of their cannons.

Several months later, Tsar Alexander I invited Kostenetsky to St. Petersburg: "How to express my gratitude, Colonel?"

"Let's make ramrods from iron instead of these made from wood, My Sovereign."

"I have no problem with introducing iron ramrods into the artillery," said the Tsar. "But where will I find more men who would be able to wield them as you did?"

After the battle of Austerlitz, Kostenetsky was awarded the Order of St. George 3rd Class and his fireworker Maslov became the recipient of the Georgievsky Cross, which—as he was a *muzhik*, in a sense a serf—prevented him from physical punishments for the rest of his life. (1) Some historians argued that two men—strong of any measure—simply could not save four guns, while being in the centre of a battle. (2) What does it matter? All of us like these miraculous feats of heroism and strength displayed by ordinary Russian soldiers. And if it did not happen at all, that is not important.

You become a general!

During the reign of Catherine II (Catherine the Great), who ruled in 1762–1796, in the year 1768 in Verevki village, in the former Konotop district in Northern Ukraine, to the family of Chernigov of provincial nobility, a son was born. He grew up like the proverbial boy from the Russian folk tale, not day by day, but hour by hour, and when he was only eleven, he was already acknowledged as the tallest lad in the district. Because young Vasily spent entire days playing at soldiers and wars, his father used to say: "You will be a general, for sure!"

Kostenetsky's stock was descended from several generations of large and powerful ancestors, living in the seventeenth century in so-called Small Russia beyond the Dnieper River. One of the family members, a very defiant man strongly dedicated to an orthodox religion, was tortured in Warsaw by whipping out his heart. From that time, the family of Kostenetsky had a heart intersected with two arrows in its coat of arms.

Under Tsar Peter I all noblemen had to serve in the army and teach their children the science of war. After Peter's death in 1725, when a son was born in a nobleman's family, he was enlisted into military service as a private, and for the years of his boyhood, he moved up the ranks year by year. Vasily was sent to the Artillery-Engineer Gentry Cadet Corps in St. Petersburg. Here, with his smart brain, good memory, and tall figure, he soon distinguished himself among other cadets as someone not to be picked on, and who had better be called "Vasily Grigorievitch." On the other hand, there was an eager beaver and a sneak, a certain man named Leschka Arakcheev, physically a teeny-weeny guy, whom Kostenetsky could not tolerate. Although he (Arakcheev) was not worth the trouble, Vasily would beat him black and blue. This was fateful in the long run.

An episode with Zubov

In 1787 a new war with Turkey began. Major-General Mikhail I. Kutuzov with his corps protected the Russian border along the Bug; then his troops were included in the action of the Ekaterinoslav army. The commander of this army was Prince G. A. Potemkin. (3) He decided to seize the Turkish fortress Ochakov on the Black Sea coast. The siege lasted a very long time, and Russian soldiers lost their lives because of many diseases. In 1888 Vasily was promoted to an ensign (officer candidate). After being involved in a number of clashes, displaying unheard of acts of heroism and strength, his fame spread throughout the army like a shot. At the Black Sea, for instance, he captured two Turkish vessels, drowning the enemies from boards with an oar. For these courageous acts and zealous service thus shown, he was summoned to Prince Grigori Potemkin.

"How do you come to be here? Did you do it from foolishness or because of puerility?"

"For my love of Russia, Your Highness," returned Kostenetsky, looking down from above.

"Now you see!" the Prince missed the presumptuous reply. "You are promoted to a second-lieutenant. Take care of yourself, young man. Be up and you will become a general!"

In 1795 Kostenetsky was promoted to the rank of lieutenant. Gathering a squad of shooters from the Cossacks of the Black Sea and under the command of Prince Potemkin, he participated in the storming and capture of the fortress Ochakov. When news of the brave lieutenant came to the capital of Russia, he was called up with Platon Zubov (4) himself, who formed a new army. At first glance, Zubov liked the lieutenant's tall figure, but as Kostenetsky sat with his full weight on an invaluable antique tabouret from Germany, which subsequently broke down to a dozen parts, he was simply stunned.

"Umoril! Teper ja verju što ty Turok kak šerpki lomal . . . Now I believe that you broke the Turks into splinters! Is your ass all right? We need more of such hulks in the Guards."

Kostenetsky was about to leave when Zubov shouted: "And you can bend a silver rouble?" The lieutenant pulled a hoary copper coin out of his pocket and without visible effort, bent it between his fingers and handed it to Zubov: "For memory's sake!" It was at the fancy-dress ball in the Winter Palace that night where Zubov showed the bent coin to all people present . . . but not to Catherine. "Why provoke providence?" he thought.

How they knew him

Around forty years after the death of Kostenetsky, one of his nephews wrote: "General Kostenetsky was a giant man renowned for his great strength. He stood well over two meters in height (six-feet seven or so), and had exceedingly broad shoulders and pleasant facial features. He was good-natured, tender-hearted, and his soldiers adored him, but he was also enormously irascible. Always firm in his convictions, he never bowed before authorities and consequently had a lot of problems in life. He loved women and women loved him; however, he never married."

> HE WAS GOOD-NATURED, TENDER-HEARTED, AND HIS SOLDIERS ADORED HIM, BUT HE WAS ALSO ENORMOUSLY IRASCIBLE.

Fifty years earlier Kostenetsky said: "My height and strength are running in my blood—I look like my father, who was *sazennyj* and broad-shouldered."

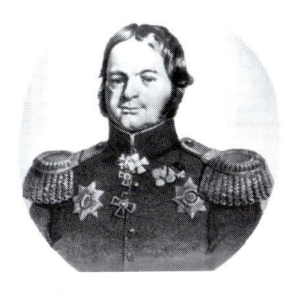

General-lieutenant V. G. Kostenetsky.

[One *sazen* in old Russian measurement units equals 213 centimeters or 7 feet.] As an artillery man he loved mathematics, knew a lot of history, and was a patriot to the highest degree and a true man of the army. He always wanted to fight and subjugate the whole of Europe for Russia. In his service record it is noted that he could speak French and German and also knew engineering, philosophy, natural law, and politics. He treated the peasants of his dominions like brothers because he grew up alongside them. Living in a village, he occasionally took off his decorated general's uniform and worked in the fields, thinking nothing of it.

Historians agreed that the general led a very unusual style of life. His idol was Generalissimus Suvorov (5) and he tried to be like him. His room was never heated. He slept on a hard leather couch, and was always uncovered and without pillows. When others tried to persuade him to take a blanket, he replied: "The soldiers during marches also have feather beds? They sleep on the ground. I am soldier as well. Last night was frosty outside so I put on a cippet. Fine, but I sweated . . . ."

Kostenetsky's nutritional habits were simple and soldierly: borscht and gruel with beef, broth or fish soup in amounts sufficient for three men. He never drank beer or wine, nor sipped tea with sugar. He always arose early and ran naked in the snow in winter. During warmer months he walked in the dew and poured buckets of ice-cold water over himself: "It is my Suvorov's morning bath!" he proclaimed proudly.

There are a great many stories and legends regarding his feats of strength. Many officers and ordinary soldiers personally witnessed Kostenetsky's uncommon might. He could break even the strongest horseshoes with his bare hands. He easily juggled with big cannonballs and was also able to carry a thick wooden beam of 25-feet long for almost 30 yards. Another time he grasped a heavy infantry musket by the barrel in an underhand grip and held it out at arm's length at shoulder level, doing this with each hand, a tremendous feat of wrist strength. Sometimes he did that with two muskets simultaneously, one in each hand (6) In battle he wielded a broad sword one-and-a-half times normal length, which was custom-made for him, instead of the

> HE ALWAYS AROSE EARLY AND RAN NAKED IN THE SNOW IN WINTER. DURING WARMER MONTHS HE WALKED IN THE DEW AND POURED BUCKETS OF ICE-COLD WATER OVER HIMSELF . . .

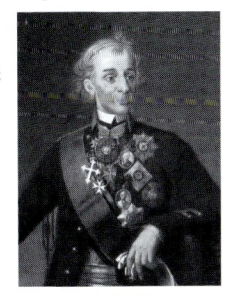

General A. Suvorov.

ordinarily-issued sabre. (7) There was also an instance where he charged the enemies with a long pipe or ramrod after his sword broke.

Once in Kiev, the general was invited to a state ball. As we already said, he was easygoing and witty, and women circled round him like wasps. This time the women intended to outsmart him. One attractive lady gave Kostenetsky a curious present, a beautiful pear made of stone. The giant in uniform balanced the pear in his hand and said: "Oh, my caring honeys! What garden is that miraculous fruit from?"

As the story goes, the General squeezed the pear in his mighty paw and it fell down into dust. "Excuse me," apologized the General. "For my taste, it is somewhat soft."

But other things had first place in Kostenetsky's life—manoeuvres, shooting practice, musters, mandatory duties, patrolling, and of course, wars. The Russian artillery was at that time—thanks to Vasily Kostenetsky, who in 1812 reached the rank of general-lieutenant—the best in the whole world. The predictions of both his father and Prince Potemkin had come true.

Getting strong, Kostenetsky-style

There is no doubt that Vasily Kostenetsky was endowed with extraordinary physical strength, which he further developed with an individual exercise regime. Firstly, the rudiments of his all-round qualities were formed with village fieldwork, wrestling, boxing, hunting, rowing, and running during his boyhood. He also enjoyed calisthenics, manual-of-arms, marches with full gear, and horseback riding—the staples of any army, and the Russians were no exception. Advancing to the rank of officer, Kostenetsky was trained in swordsmanship, both on the ground and on a galloping horse, and certainly undertook quite a few personal combats with both sabre and sword. It is necessary to add that because of Kostenetsky's huge weight, his horses were soon worn out or ill.

> **He then laid his hand on a big round iron shot weighing about 20 lb. (9 kg), and began tossing it from hand to hand.**

When the General was in the mood, he sociably chatted with his soldiers. One of them asked: "How did you get so strong, my commander?"

"Life of a soldier and exercises with cannonballs," replied Kostenetsky, who was in his fifties at that time.

He then laid his hand on a big round iron shot weighing about 20 lb. (9 kg), and began tossing it from hand to hand. He gradually increased the speed of motion, tossing the ball with a straight arm overhead, where it made a wide arc from the right side to the left, and finally catching the plummeting weight on the palm of his left hand. All the soldiers standing around him gasped in amazement.

Next, bending forward at the waist and holding the ball with two hands between his legs, Kostenetsky swung the weight upward to arm's length overhead, loosening his grip in the process. He waited, standing erect, and then gently caught the falling ball in his hands which were above his head. The general also performed various forms of crucifixes, unilaterally or with both arms outstretched to the sides, with one or more balls lying on his palms.

"You must put a lot of effort while working on my exercises," continued Kostenetsky. "As a little boy I had a leather ball made into which I poured peas. It was my toy for years. I would toss it up and catch it, either lying or standing, even with friends in village. Later I needed a bigger ball, filled with peas and lead shots—it weighed ten pounds!—and my exercising started again. I exercised every day."

Aftermath

Forty years passed and times changed for the worse. Leschka Arakcheev, now count Alexey Andreevitch Arakcheev (8) and the head of the War Council of the State Department, never forgot the insults that he got from Kostenetsky in the corps. Subsequently, the military career of Kostenetsky under Arakcheev came to a halt. The hero from Austerlitz was dispatched to remote parts of Russia, disregarded in gradation, and simply left in service. In 1812 he commanded the whole artillery of the Russian army, futilely waiting for praise. The general became reserved and distrustful as he did not receive any further rewards but was the object of Arakcheev's revenge.

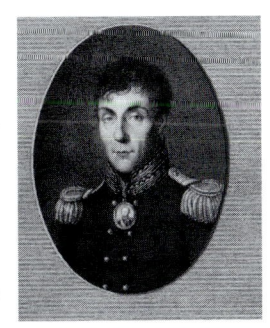

A. A. Arakcheev.
Photos courtesy of Joseph Svub.

Kostenetsky was the recipient of the Order of St. Vladimir 2nd Class; instead of an order of a higher class, he was "rewarded" with the same order.

General Kostenetsky was doomed to meet a sad end: he did not fall in battle but died on a hospital bed. What could not be brought about by shots or sabres was brought about by one small germ of vibrio cholerae. (9) He passed away on 6 July 1831, approaching the age of sixty-three.

From the *Encyclopedic Dictionary* of F. A. Brockhaus and I. A. Efron, the entry reads: "Kostenetsky Vasily Grigorievitch, general-lieutenant, he studied in the Artillery-Engineer Gentry Cadet Corps. After the battle of Borodino he commanded the whole artillery of the Russian army and took important part in actions at Tarutine, Malo-Yaroslavets, and Krasny; in 1813–1814 he participated in the main battles." (Vol. XVI, page 389). And this phrase is written in *Codex Regius* from Iceland (1270): "I know only one, what stands forever—a legend of a late." The Russians long cherished the memory of General Kostenetsky. M

Main sources:
1. Lavrov, Valentin: *Istoki bogatyrstva*, Moscow 1989 (an original print).
2. Wikipedia: "Battle of Austerlitz"

Notes:
1. The Russian army in the 1800s had many characteristics of ancient organisation. There was no permanent formation above the regimental level; senior officers were largely recruited from aristocratic circles, and the Russian soldier, in line with eighteenth century practices, was regularly beaten and punished "to instill discipline." Nevertheless, the Russians did have fine artillery, manned by soldiers who regularly fought hard to prevent their pieces from falling into enemy hands.

2. In 1802, a commission for reorganizing the artillery was formed under the chairmanship of A. A. Arakcheev. The commission worked out a new weapons system: a 12-pounder cannon with a caliber of 120 mm, a barrel weighing 800 kg (1,760 lb.) and a 640-kg (1,408-lb.) carriage, etc. Special implements were used, such as a cleaning rod (*bannik*) with rammer or a bristle brush. The ramrod was a device used to push the projectile up against the gunpowder. For moving cannons, the rear crosspiece of the gun was put over the vertical pin and secured with chains. For a 12-pounder cannon, six horses were harnessed. The total weight of a 12-pounder for a campaign was 1,700 kg (3,740 lb.).

3. This is not the same person as Major-General J. A. Potemkin, who began his military career in the Guards and became a colonel at the age of 23, with his first big military experience being the battle of Austerlitz in 1805. The Potemkin of our article, His Serene Highness Prince Grigori A. Potemkin (1739–1791) was a Russian general field marshal, statesman, and favourite of Catherine II. After studying at the University of Moscow, he enlisted in the horse guards, where he received the rank of second-lieutenant. He participated in the Palace revolution in 1762, which ousted Peter III and enthroned Catherine II. The Empress needed reliable assistants and appreciated Potemkin's energy and organizational abilities. He is primarily remembered for his efforts to civilise the wild steppes of Southern Ukraine.

4. Platon A. Zubov (1767–1822) was the last of Catherine II's favourites and the most powerful man in the Russian Empire during the last years of her reign. When they met, Catherine was over 60 and Zubov was just 22. Zubov, however, contrived to establish a stronghold on Catherine's affections. In seven years he was made a count and then a prince of the Holy Roman Empire. Upon Potemkin's death she appointed him successor as the Governor-General of New Russia. F. Rostopchin wrote in 1795: "Count Zubov is everything here. There is no other will but his. His power is greater than that of Potemkin . . . The Empress keeps repeating that he is the greatest genius the history of Russia has known."

5. Alexander Vasilyevitch Suvorov (1729–1800), one of the few great generals in history who never lost a battle, was famed for his manual *The Science of Victory* and noted for the sayings, "Train hard, fight easy," "Perish yourself, but rescue your comrade," and "The bullet is a fool, the bayonet is a fine chap." Perhaps his most famous feat occurred when Suvorov had passed with his army through the snow-capped Alps in 1799—he was almost 80 years old. For this marvel of strategic retreat, unheard of since the time of Hannibal, Suvorov became the fourth generalissimus of the Russian Empire.

6. The firearms in the Russian army were not uniform. For example, the 1808 pattern infantry musket was 145 cm (57 in.) long and its weight (without the bayonet) was 4.47 kg (9.8 lb).

7. The Russian heavy cavalry in 1812 had several models of broad swords. For dragoons it was the 1806 model with the blade 89 cm (35 in.) long and up to 3.8 cm wide. It weighed 1.65 kg (3.6 lb.).

8. A. A. Arakcheev (1769–1834), count, statesman, military commander and artillery general, became commandant of St. Petersburg in 1796, one of the highest and closest officials connected to the Tsar. In 1808–1810 he held the posts of Minister of War and Infantry-Artillery Inspector General. After the war, Alexander I's trust in Arakcheev increased so that he confided to him the execution of the highest commands not only in the military, but also in civil matters. He was also known for his repressive domestic policies as commander of the Internal Security Forces, and for his desire to maintain a pre-Napoleonic status quo in Europe. From 1816 he virtually ran domestic state policy and personally presented reports on all state affairs to the Tsar.

9. The Asiatic cholera, originating in Bengal, India, began its deadly march around the world in 1817. It swept across Russia and Poland and reached Berlin in 1831. Every twentieth Russian and thirtieth Pole died in 1830.

Sumo
Strength

Ken Best

I've had a fascination with sumo since I was a teenager, when I became a practitioner of karate. As an avid student of the martial arts, I was surprised to learn that sumo was the oldest form of Japanese combat. From then on, it remained a favorite topic of mine throughout my adult life, particularly when I became a strength athlete.

At first I was a skinny 20-year-old, with next to no equipment and minimal funds, looking for a method of putting on as much muscular bulk and strength as I could. Naturally, I began to research the bulk-building methods of the sumo. After all, Asian wrestlers proved long ago that combining training with excess calorie consumption and rest could produce huge gains in size and strength.

I recently went to Japan on a cultural tour with my son and his language class. I had some idea of Japanese culture from my martial arts background, but experiencing it in person was all I had hoped for and more. Unfortunately, I was unable to visit a sumo stable and witness for myself their training, but over the years I've collected much information on the subject. When I returned to Australia, I was still in the mood for all things Japanese, so I wrote this article to share with my fellow MILO readers the training techniques and bulk-building methods of the sumo wrestlers. But first, some background information on Japan is necessary in order to understand the fascinating sport it spawned.

Japan is a culture of contrasts. It produces cutting-edge technology for the world's benefit, but holds on to its traditions as though it would crumble without them. Japanese people are deeply religious, and many of their traditions stem from Shinto or Buddhist beliefs. Japan's history is defined by centuries of war and martial rule. Shoguns controlled much of the country through forceful reign, commanding their many samurai warriors to do their bidding. The emperor was only a royal figurehead until the shogun gave the power of rule back to the royal family at the end of the Edo period, thereby ending years of internal strife and bringing peace to the country.

Despite the influences of the western world, Japanese people continue to practice many of their traditions. Rituals, such as the tea ceremony and calligraphy, remain unchanged from the way they were performed centuries ago. Japanese people are by and large very patriotic and hold dear the ways of old. Traditional clothing is still worn at formal ceremonies, such as weddings, funerals, and religious celebrations. Martial arts are practiced by men, women, and children alike. Geisha still provide their special services and are in much demand. Japan's national sport, sumo, is contested just as it has been for over a hundred years and its origins date back long before that.

The sport of sumo is believed to be at least a thousand years old. Many experts believe it could be even more ancient than that, and agree that it stemmed from Shinto rituals to celebrate the end of the harvest. Rice farmers would take on each other in the most basic of wrestling matches to bring good luck to the victor in the next harvest. Most of the techniques, rules, costumes, and victory rituals remain today, making it one of the oldest and most colorful of sports. Victory in sumo is achieved when one wrestler pushes the other out of the ring (called the *dohyo*) or causes the other wrestler to make contact with the clay with any part of his body except for the soles of the feet.

A day in the life of a sumo wrestler or *rikishi* (meaning strong samurai) starts early, around 6 A.M. Upon rising, he immediately commences training. Training is divided into two sessions: contact rehearsal and exercises (solo training). Contact rehearsal is done first and takes various forms, such as knockout sparring, where the victor continues to wrestle new opponents until eliminated; rushing practice, where a senior stands in the middle of the ring and allows juniors to collide with him; and partner training, in which bouts are repeated against the same opponent. Injuries and concussions are common. Contact practice goes until mid-morning, after which the wrestler moves on to solo exercises.

The exercises the wrestlers perform during solo training form the basis for their strength- and bulk-building program. It should come as no surprise to MILO readers that central to their methods is the deep knee bend or squat. Wrestlers perform hundreds of bodyweight squats as well as high-repetition squats holding a heavy round stone not unlike an Atlas stone (only not quite so heavy). They also typically do a hundred or more *shiko*, or high stomps, where they smash each foot onto the clay. They do other leg-strengthening movements, such as duck walks and partner carries, and sit for long periods of time in a full-squat position as they are required to do so prior to each bout.

Wrestlers train their upper bodies with high-repetition push-ups with bodyweight or with a wrestler sitting on their shoulders (a favorite exercise of judoka as well), and high-repetition smacks into a teppo pole, a large wooden post. Stretching is also done, the most common stretch (and the most painful to witness) being the *matawari*, or thigh split. Trainees sit in a split-legged position and lean forward to touch their noses to the ground. If they can't get low enough, a senior *rikishi* pushes down on their necks, forcing them to the completed posture.

Once the training session is finished, the wrestlers are free to do calisthenics, weight training, and cool-down exercises if they have the energy. Most modern sumo supplement their training with weights, and the powerlifts are popular. Senior *rikishi* perform barbell squats, bench presses, deadlifts, and

> RICE FARMERS WOULD TAKE ON EACH OTHER IN THE MOST BASIC OF WRESTLING MATCHES TO BRING GOOD LUCK TO THE VICTOR IN THE NEXT HARVEST.

> IT SHOULD COME AS NO SURPRISE TO MILO READERS THAT CENTRAL TO THEIR METHODS IS THE DEEP KNEE BEND OR SQUAT.

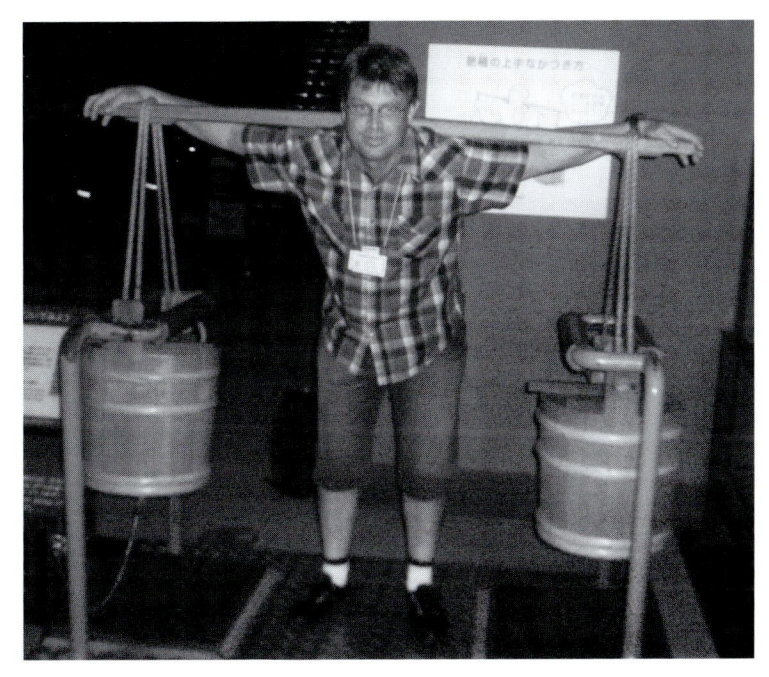

Ken Best gets under an old yoke at the Edo-Tokyo Museum: "The yoke I'm shouldering is what the farmers used to carry human waste in from the city to the farm to use as fertilizer. Each bucket when full weighed about 15 kg. The farmers carried the yoke for miles and did it every day. Talk about endurance!"
Billy Best photo.

other heavy free-weight exercises for limited sets and repetitions in a systematic way, similar to modern powerlifting programs. It is safe to say that many *rikishi* possess the strength and power of national and world-class powerlifters and strongman competitors.

Let's examine sumo training in detail and highlight why it works so well. Squats are the cornerstone not only of sumo wrestlers' training but also that of many other athletes. Why? The answer is obvious to a MILO reader: Heavy, high-repetition squats have proven time and again that they can transform a skinny, weak "before" specimen into a strong, muscular, and healthy "after." Even bodyweight squats can cause such a transformation if coupled with the right diet. Young *rikishi* start with bodyweight squats and add stone squats as they mature and gain weight. Senior *rikishi* perform barbell squats and manage to handle hundreds of pounds in this exercise. There is no question that this approach to strength-and-bulk training works. Senior *rikishi* commonly reach the 400-plus pound bodyweight mark.

Leg lifts and stomps supplement their leg training and are more specific to their sport. The pre-bout ritual requires each wrestler to stomp the clay to ward off evil spirits. Stomping also strengthens the legs and hips for fighting in the *dohyo*. Steve Justa talks about this type of strength training in his book *Rock Iron Steel* and calls it G-force training. He states that it builds speed-strength and stopping-strength and is great for fighting skills. I agree and so do thousands of *rikishi*. Steve also describes sumo wrestlers' leg training as consisting of heavy pulls and drags. These exercises build the strength needed to pull, drag and push their opponents around the *dohyo*.

Push-ups are done in high numbers by young *rikishi* and usually with another wrestler sitting or lying on their backs. Senior *rikishi* like to do bench presses with free weights. As a matter of fact, Chiyonofuji (the Wolf), arguably the greatest *yokozuna* (grand champion) in the history of the sport and my personal favorite, used the bench press to rehabilitate a dislocated left shoulder and went on to be the second most successful *yokozuna*, with 29 championship wins to his credit. He was one of the first *rikishi* to adopt weight training to build muscle and speed, and many *rikishi* have since followed his lead. Open-handed slaps on the teppo pole build the same kind of strength in the wrestlers' hands, arms and shoulders as do the leg stomps for the legs, and are specific to pushing and slapping an opponent out of the *dohyo*.

Back work involves a lot of wrestling moves, such as pulling, lifting, and throwing opponents. This condensed work builds the arms, traps and lower backs of the *rikishi* to phenomenal levels. Modern *rikishi* also supplement their back training with deadlifts, curls, and rows with free weights. As mentioned above, some wrestlers train with odd objects and do sled drags, stone lifts and the like. One of the most popular techniques in sumo is called *tsuri-dashi*, which means lift-out. With a strong two-handed grip on the rear of the opponent's belt, the attacker lifts him up in the air and carries him over the straw ridge for the win. Naturally this move requires a great deal of body power to execute, and it relies on a strong grip and upper back.

> HE WAS ONE OF THE FIRST *RIKISHI* TO ADOPT WEIGHT TRAINING TO BUILD MUSCLE AND SPEED, AND MANY *RIKISHI* HAVE SINCE FOLLOWED HIS LEAD.

Core strength is built with high-repetition frog kicks and sit-ups, as well as twisting and throwing movements against an opponent. Naturally, sumo wrestlers don't train to show their six-packs, but their core strength is obviously good, considering they wrestle large opponents on a daily basis. Many people dismiss sumo wrestlers as just fat men in shiny nappies bellying each other around the ring until someone falls out. Nothing could be further from the truth. Sumo wrestlers are professional athletes in every respect. They train, eat, and live the sport. They are covered in fat, but this is to their advantage because sumos need to have a low centre of gravity, and a large belly helps in this regard.

However, underneath the layer of fat is a very strong, powerfully-built athlete . . . and it is not necessary to carry huge amounts of weight. Chiyonofuji, at the peak of his fighting career, weighed only 122 kg and had very little bodyfat. Also, Musashimaru, a Hawaiian wrestler and *yokozuna*, had a bodyfat percentage of around 20 throughout his career. There are no weight divisions in sumo, so it makes sense to a wrestler that to be competitive, he should weigh as much as possible. But beyond a certain point, weight by itself is a disadvantage. With the

> HOWEVER, UNDERNEATH THE LAYER OF FAT IS A VERY STRONG, POWERFULLY-BUILT ATHLETE . . . AND IT IS NOT NECESSARY TO CARRY HUGE AMOUNTS OF WEIGHT.

inclusion of weight training in the wrestlers' programs, many *rikishi* became stronger, quicker and more muscular, and hence more successful.

Upon my return to Australia, I discovered I had gained 5 kg whilst away and weighed 100 kg. I hadn't trained for two weeks, and I had overindulged in a wide range of delicious Japanese food. It was the beginning of November and summer was just around the corner. I wanted to lose the weight I gained in Japan whilst holding onto as much muscle as possible. In light of my trip to Japan, I decided to modify my training to include the exercises described in this article, and experiment with them to see what affect they would have on my physique and fitness.

C1 (Circuit 1):
- bodyweight squats x 100
- sit-ups x 50
- push-ups x 50
- front/rear neck holds x 30 sec.
- pull-ups x 5
- CoC grippers, Trainer x 20, No. 1 x 5

If I didn't get all reps in the first circuit, I'd do another until rep targets were met.

C2 (Circuit 2):
- sandbag squats, 50 kg x 20
- leg raises x 20
- dips x 5
- neck harness, 20 kg x 10
- chin-ups x 5
- CoC grippers No. 1.5 x 5

I increased the abdominal, neck, and grip work as I went.

C3 (Circuit 3):
- stomps x 10 each leg
- side bends x 10 using cables
- hand slaps against tree trunk x 10 each hand
- manual side neck work x 10
- cable curls x 8
- CoC grippers, No. 2 x max
- one set each direction on the wrist roller, 20 kg

I trained three days a week, usually Monday, Wednesday, and Friday. Each training session I began with a circuit of bodyweight exercises (C_1). Monday was my heavy day so after C_1, I completed C_2 and C_3 with minimal rest between circuits. The sandbag I used for the squats weighed 50 kg. Chins and dips were done for reps without weights attached. The cable curls were performed with IronMind's Fabled Cables and seven bands.

I worked through each circuit without rest. I added 10 reps each week on squats, 5 reps on push-ups, 1 rep on chins/dips, and 5 stomps/slaps each limb. Wednesday was my light day so I only completed C_1, followed by a few rehab exercises for my back injury. Friday was a medium day so I did C_1 and C_3. Grip work was completed using Captains of Crush® Grippers and the Twist Yo' Wrist wrist roller. I followed each session with a half hour of cardio in the form of swimming.

As you can see, there were no exercises done with free weights—for two reasons. Firstly, I wanted to lose bodyfat whilst maintaining muscle mass. I felt that a routine with mostly bodyweight exercises would best accomplish this goal. Secondly, I wanted to train the way traditional sumo wrestlers would have trained, just for the experience. I could have modified the above routine by substituting barbell squats, bench presses, and deadlifts or rows for the exercises in C_2 if I had wanted to add muscular bodyweight and strength without losing bodyfat (in much the same way as modern sumo train). Maybe the next time I tackle this routine, I'll substitute free weights and report on the results.

I followed this routine for 10 weeks. I lost 6 kg of bodyweight, and judging from the mirror, it was all bodyfat. I maintained my muscle mass and became more muscular and leaner. My conditioning went through the roof, based on my energy levels at the end of the working week. I slept like a log every night and my mood was much improved even though it was the silly season and the Christmas/New Year week was upon us. I didn't change my diet apart from eating more salads and fruit. On one weekend day each week, I would get out into the gully and do some strength lifting with odd objects, such as rock lifts and throws, car pushes, and log drags, to simulate wrestling a heavy opponent.

> THE SECRET TO SUMO WRESTLERS' MASSIVE WEIGHT GAINS HAS TO DO WITH WHAT THEY EAT, WHEN THEY EAT, AND HOW MUCH THEY EAT.

It appears from the above results that sumo training doesn't work when the goal is to gain muscular bodyweight. My training was only slightly different from sumo wrestlers. For a start, sumos train for hours every day. Their training involves a lot of wrestling with heavy opponents, and they use heavier weights and bodyweight in their solo training than I did. The choice of exercises wasn't the issue. I followed a strict, calorie-controlled diet because I wanted to lose bodyfat. I ate small meals every two to three hours. These meals consisted of lean protein, salad, and vegetables or fruit. My diet was high-protein and low-fat, with almost no carbs. My diet was the determining factor in my weight-loss efforts. If we examine the diet of the sumos, you can see that it also determines their rate of weight gain.

The secret to sumo wrestlers' massive weight gains has to do with what they eat, when they eat, and how much they eat. They eat only twice a day, but at each sitting they consume huge amounts of food. They don't eat breakfast for practical reasons, as they would lose their stomach contents once they began training. After training, however, they are ravenous and sit down to bowls and bowls of food. They eat a stew called *chanko-nabe*, which consists of meat, seafood, eggs, tofu and vegetables, coupled with many bowls of white rice and copious quantities of beer and *sake* (rice wine). They then sleep all afternoon to aid digestion and recovery. They eat again at night and often consume more alcohol at their numerous guest appearances and sponsorship commitments.

Unfortunately, this type of diet also leads to many health problems, the worst being diabetes. The sumos' excessive diet is high in carbohydrates and calories eaten over a long time, which plays havoc with their metabolism and insulin levels. Coupled with their bodyweight, this situation leads to diabetes at a young age and a host of other illnesses, such as heart disease, hypertension, and liver disease. As a result, the average lifespan of a *rikishi* is 60 years, and they retire from the sport before they turn 40. A senior *rikishi* is lucky to retire healthy, with minimal injuries. This trend is changing, however, as more *rikishi* rely on heavy weight training rather than the *chanko* pot to gain weight.

If you would like to try the sumo's approach to strength training, give my routine a go. You can couple it with any other sport you participate in. If you're a wrestler or martial artist, it could be just what you're looking for. After all, sumo is one of the oldest martial sports and believed to be the basis for all the other Japanese martial arts. Wrestling in and of itself is good strength training and builds a unique type of whole-body power. Adding this type of training to the mix can only help your performance on the mat. If you have minimal equipment, a tight budget, or limited training space, this routine may be just what you need. Do the routine as written if you want to lose fat weight, or substitute your favorite free-weight exercises for strength and muscle gain.

Some words of caution are in order. You should couple your routine with a high-protein, high-calorie diet if you want to gain. I don't recommend force-feeding yourself at two meals unless you are particularly lean. You don't need a lot of alcohol either. Spread your meals into four to six servings and consume them throughout the day, or use a protein powder in place of two or three meals. Get plenty of rest and sleep, and train hard. You know the formula: train, eat, sleep . . . Also, stomps, slaps and other sudden-impact training can be hard on your bones and joints if you're not used to doing them. Start slowly and work into it.

> IT WOULD BE WRONG TO IGNORE OR DISMISS THEIR METHODS AS OLD-FASHIONED AND OBSOLETE.

Sumo wrestlers have had over a thousand years of experience in gaining functional bodyweight for use in their sport. Until the late 1980s, they used little more than bodyweight, odd objects and partner-assisted movements to accomplish this feat. When they discovered weight training, they added it to the mix without discarding their traditional ways. I don't believe they did this just out of a sense of duty or to honor their culture, but because their methods worked. It would be wrong to ignore or dismiss their methods as old-fashioned and obsolete. The success and staying power of the sport of sumo in history says otherwise. I look forward to the future of sumo, as modern training approaches and information sources permeate the sport and produce healthier, stronger and better athletes. MILO is such a source.

Sources:

1. Randall J. Strossen, "Asian Wrestlers: Bulging with Basics," *Hardgainer* Magazine, Volume 1, Number 4 (January 1990).
2. Angela Patmore, *The Giants of Sumo* (London: Queen Anne Press, 1990).
3. Andy Adams and Clyde Newton, *Sumo* (London: The Hamilton Publishing Group, 1989).
4. Steve Justa, *Rock Iron Steel: The Book of Strength* (Nevada City, CA: IronMind Enterprises, 1998).

IRON FILINGS
Randall J. Strossen, Ph.D. | *Publisher & Editor-in-chief*

Magnus Samuelsson is the first person to win World's Strongest Man and *Dancing With the Stars*, and the media attention he has been getting is "phenomenal." Sure, he's a World's Strongest Man winner as well as someone who closes the No. 3 Captains of Crush Gripper with consummate ease and has "no fear of the No. 4," but for a guy who'd "never taken a dance step before this," Magnus Samuelsson has done himself proud by winning *Dancing With the Stars* in Sweden. "It's been a long road," Magnus Samuelsson told IronMind, "four months of 4 or 5 hours a day practicing. It's going to be a relief to get back in the gym."

Magnus said he was getting tremendous exposure from being in the contest: "Sweden has a population of 8 million people and each week 2 million watch this show. It's like winning World's Strongest Man every week." And speaking of winning World's Strongest Man, don't rule out the possibility of seeing Magnus Samuelsson active in strongman on a selective basis later this year.

Since his dance floor victory, Samuelsson said he is receiving "requests for 15 or 20 shows a day," taking him from prominence in the strength world to much broader markets: "It is quite remarkable that because of dancing, something I'd never done before, all of this has happened." **M**

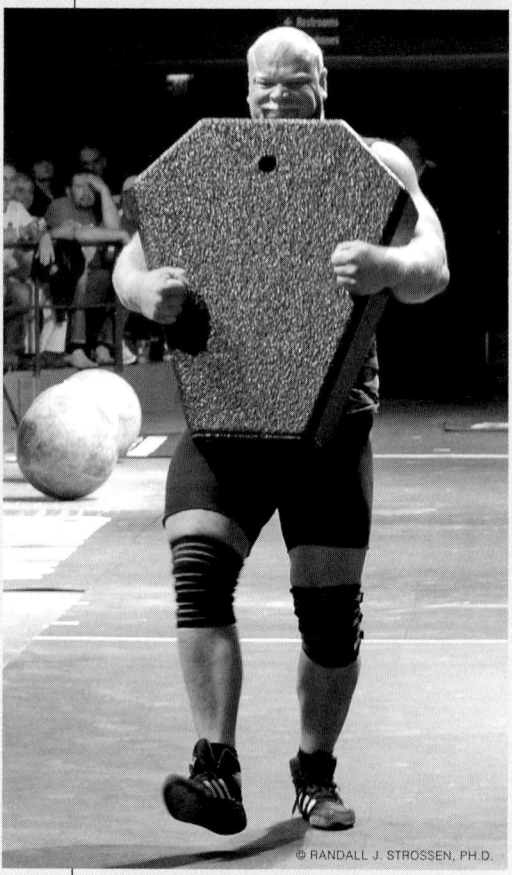

When you're a World's Strongest Man winner, this is how you cross train for *Dancing With the Stars*. Ask Magnus Samuelsson, the first (and to date the only) person ever to win both contests.
Randall J. Strossen photo.

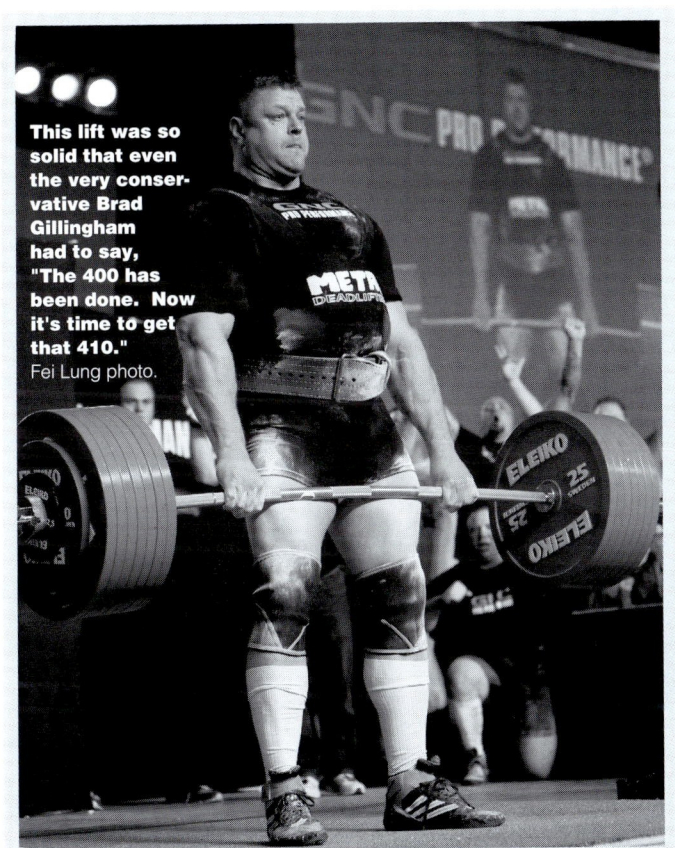

This lift was so solid that even the very conservative Brad Gillingham had to say, "The 400 has been done. Now it's time to get that 410."
Fei Lung photo.

Brad Gillingham is a two-time International Powerlifting Federation (IPF) world champion, so don't think he lifts in the masters' because he couldn't lift anything heavy when he was a mere stripling. For his competitors, at least, the problem is that the older Brad Gillingham gets, the more he's lifting.

Pulling that 390-kg deadlift at last year's IPF Men's World Championships was a pretty big deal, especially considering that Brad Gillingham was 41 years old at the time. Rather than resting on his laurels, the IPF Hall-of-Famer was back for more this year as he totaled 1057.5 kg to win the IPF World Masters' Championships, breaking his own masters' world records in the deadlift and in the total. That total represented a 5-kg increase over what Brad did at the 2007 IPF Men's World Championships, but the even bigger news was that Brad's 395-kg deadlift is a lifetime PR.

We had to ask Brad whether he was thinking of hitting a 400-kg deadlift and there was no waffle in his answer: "That would be the goal," he said. "I'm too ornery to quit." And if you wanted to be on hand to see it, we recommended that it would be a good idea to be at the 2009 Arnold, where the USAPL was hosting multiple powerlifting events, and Brad Gillingham was scheduled to be among the competitors.

With his string of successes, Brad Gillingham already had plenty of incentive to keep this roll alive, but how this for frosting on the cake: Brad was in the number-one position on the 2008 IPF World rankings, causing the typically taciturn Gillingham to say, "The old man showed the young guys that he is still around!"

Fast forward to the Arnold and Gilly made good, yet again: his first 400-kg deadlift! **M**

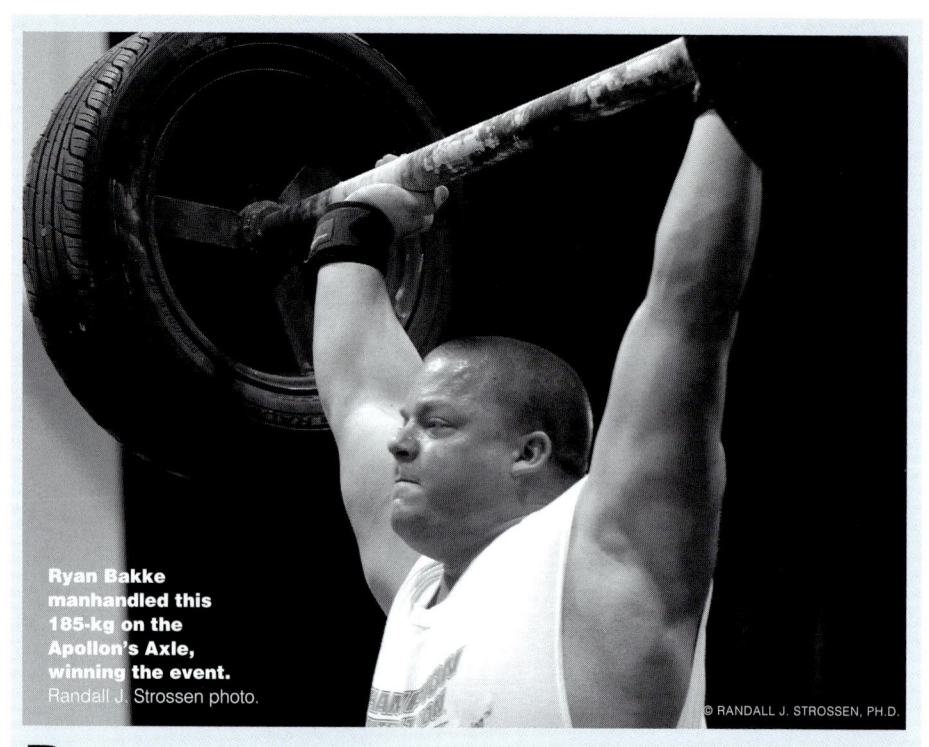

Ryan Bakke manhandled this 185-kg on the Apollon's Axle, winning the event.
Randall J. Strossen photo.

Ryan Bakke kicked off the Gaspari Nutrition All-American Strongman Challenge by setting a new world record in the Apollon's Axle overhead lift, getting 185 kg from the ground to arm's length overhead at the FitExpo held in January 2009 in Los Angeles, California. Brian Shaw and Pete Konradt tied for second in this event, both making 180 kg. Marshall White overpowered the rest of the field on the dotFIT Crucifix Hold, easily winning the event. Pete Konradt was second, followed by Kevin Nee. The third event bore the imprint of contest organizer Odd Haugen, as the farmer's walk went from heavy to heavier to heaviest in a three-implement, three-stage event that started with a pair of 325-lb. suitcases, next used a pair of 385-lb. cylinders, and then finished with an 880-lb. frame. Brian Shaw won, Nick Best was second, and Travis Ortmayer was third.

Brian Shaw treated day one's very strong performance as a warm-up and on day two he lowered the boom, winning in a most impressive manner. "Brian Shaw's performance was nothing short of spectacular," Odd Haugen told *MILO*. Brian jump started his day by winning the Axle deadlift, hitting 385 kg, and then Nick Best won the Super Yoke carry. The final event was the Stones of Strength and even with all the top stone lifters in this contest, only two competitors succeeded in loading all six stones: Brian Shaw (who won the event) and Nick Best. The final placings were: 1. Brian Shaw, 2. Nick Best, 3. Travis Ortmayer, 4. Marshall White, 5. Kevin Nee. Unfortunately, Kevin Nee tore his biceps on the deadlift, but he persevered though the yoke, although he could not do the stones. **M**

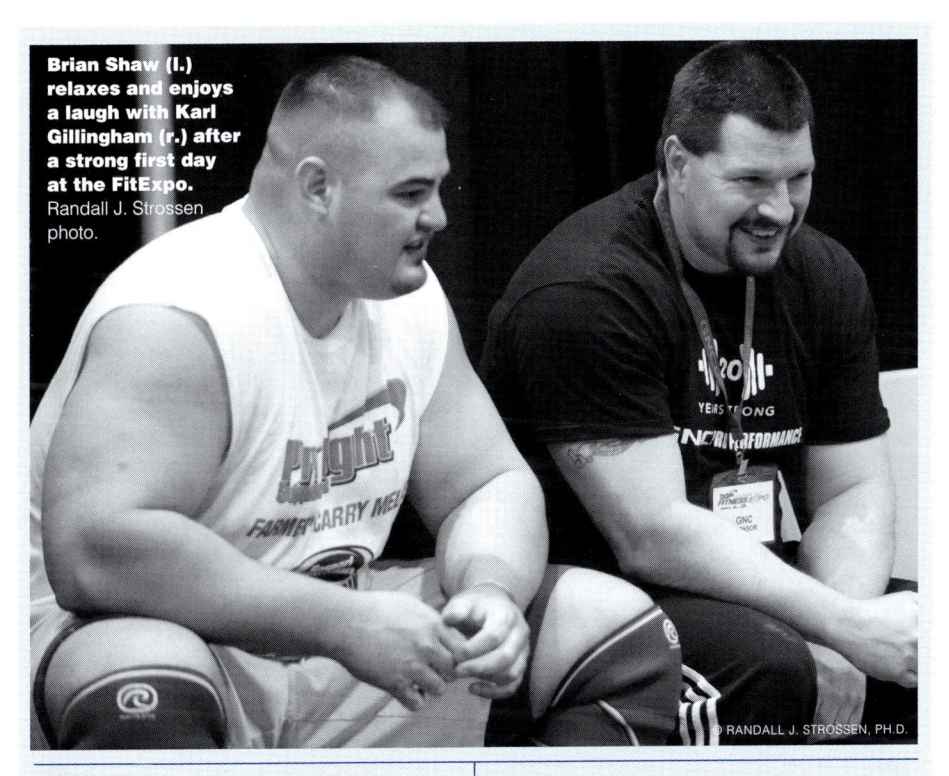

Brian Shaw (l.) relaxes and enjoys a laugh with Karl Gillingham (r.) after a strong first day at the FitExpo.
Randall J. Strossen photo.

When the February–March issue of *Business Week's SmallBiz* magazine hit the newsstands, one of the articles inside featured IronMind. Focusing on Captains of Crush® Grippers and noting IronMind's marketing acumen, the article presented the small California business and one of its signature products to an audience that might never have known how addictive strength training—especially on Captains of Crush Grippers—can be. IronMind founder and president Randall Strossen said, "I was quite surprised and immensely flattered when *Business Week* writer Louise Lee called—this was big news at IronMind." If you can't get your hands on a hard copy of the magazine, you can read the article, "Get a Grip" online: http://www.businessweek.com/magazine/content/09_62/s0902021045210.htm.

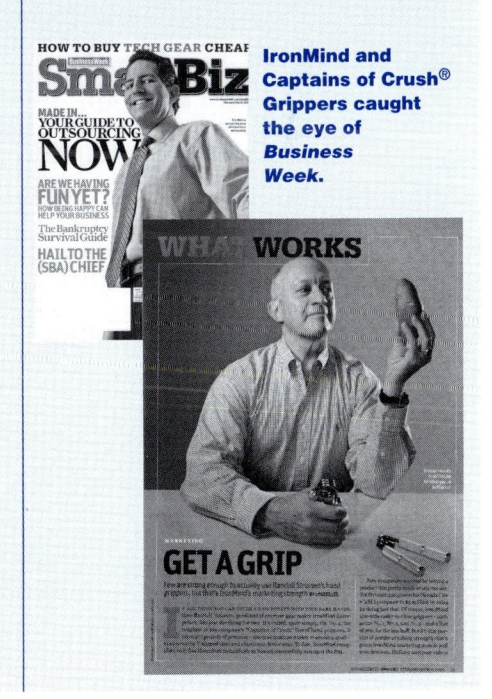

M

IronMind and Captains of Crush® Grippers caught the eye of *Business Week*.

Derek Poundstone decimated the field on the Circus Dumbbell, leapfrogging over Mikhail Koklyaev to claim the 2009 Arnold Strongman title.
Randall J. Strossen photo.

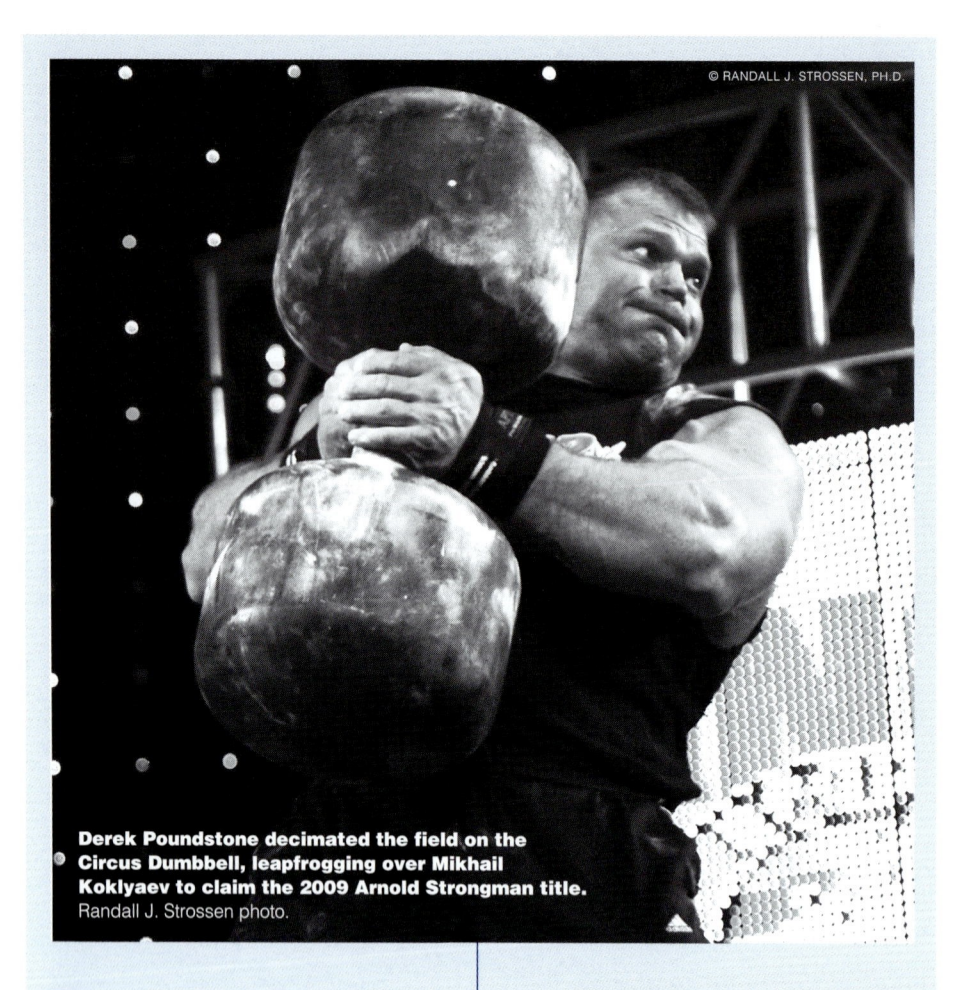

Derek Poundstone won the Arnold Strongman contest in Columbus, Ohio, the first to hold the title after the five-year winning streak by Zydrunas Savickas. Mikhail Koklyaev was second and Travis Ortmayer was third. Poundstone came into the final event, the Circus Dumbbell, trailing Koklyaev by two points, so to win the contest, he would have to beat Koklyaev; and at least one other competitor would have to place between himself and the Russian strongman. Poundstone left no doubt that he was playing for keeps as he banged out 15 reps, 6 more than the top performance up to that point. Koklyaev needed 10 reps to win, but he had to settle for 8, which dropped him from first to second place overall. Travis Ortmayer made 9 reps, moving him from a tie for fourth place to third place overall in the final standings.

M

After the Arnold Sports Festival, where they starred in the IronMind Invitational, the German men's Olympic weightlifting team was warmly welcomed in Chicago for a few days before returning home. Chicago has a lot going for it and the Olympic sport of weightlifting is part of the picture. Whether you look back at the city's deep roots in the sport or peer into its future—which includes its status as a 2016 Olympic candidate city—Chicago offers the perfect setting for welcoming the German men's Olympic weightlifting team. Mike Gattone was tapped to be the liaison for this visit by the German Weightlifting Federation's elite delegation, a group that included gold medalist Matthias Steiner; Germany's top weightlifting coach, Frank Mantek; and a former world champion and a world record holder in the sport, Marc Huster.

Currently working as the High Performance and Coaching Education Director for USA Weightlifting, Gattone has a standout background that includes serving as Weightlifting Competition Director at the 1996 Olympic Games and later working as the assistant strength and conditioning coach for the Chicago Bulls. "We are fortunate to have someone with Mike Gattone's track record and commitment to weightlifting on the ground and ready to run in Chicago," said Randall Strossen, who made the introduction, asking Gattone if he could spearhead the visit by the German weightlifting delegation. Gattone agreed and he arranged training sessions and a dinner honoring the guests, as well as a series of meetings and appearances around Chicago.

The visit itself was on a roll from the moment the German delegation collected its luggage and looking outside, mused about who the limo was for . . . and it turned out that it was for them, courtesy of 2016, the entity dedicated to bringing the 2016 Olympics to Chicago.

On Monday, the group trained at WCS/Gattone Sports Performance in Buffalo Grove. One of the things that caught Mike's eye was the emphasis on both push presses and regular standing presses, two movements that head coach Frank Mantek values highly. Mike said the Germans also did pulls and that they do them in two styles: the conventional way based on what they can do in the full lifts and also heavier, as in the snatch or clean deadlift and shrug that Jim Schmitz advocates. The German lifters are also used to following their workouts with massage or sauna and a cold plunge or a jacuzzi.

The next day, training was at the University of Illinois–Chicago, where their workouts included squats. Mike said that when he asked Matthias Steiner who had stronger legs—Matthias or Ronny Weller—Matthias said it was no contest . . . Ronny was a better squatter. The Germans never go below triples for squats and they might use reps as high as 8. Mike said that head coach Frank Mantek was quick to disavow any ideas that he is a guru, but said that instead, he emphasizes good technique and a periodized training system that can draw from a menu of 15 exercises.

The German delegation also visited the Lindbloom Academy in Chicago's South Side, and Matthias Steiner, speaking in English, asked the students, "Did you ever hear the speech 'I have a dream?' Well, I had a dream, to win an Olympic gold medal," at which point he pulled out his gold medal and the students went wild. Frank Mantek followed, speaking in German translated by Dr. Christian Baumgartner, and he told the students, "There is an Olympic champion in this school!"

Dinner was at Gibson's, the top-end, see-and-be-seen Chicago steakhouse, where they took a picture of Matthias Steiner for their wall.

Mike also said that the German delegation went over to the Sears Tower, and Frank Mantek returned with a big photo of Chicago's own, U.S. President Barack Obama! M

ASC's Dione Wessels and IronMind's Randall Strossen are teaming up to put grip contests front and center by featuring them at American Strongman Corporation's "Live" events across the country.

"Testing your grip strength provides a natural challenge and it's fun, so Dione and I thought, why not take advantage of the 'Live' platform to showcase the IronMind Grip Challenge," said Strossen. "We wanted to feature events that are universally-known, with well-established standards of excellence. The two events we are going with are the Rolling Thunder®, for maximum weight, and Captains of Crush® Grippers. We're running grippers the way stones are done in strongman: a tougher gripper always wins, but reps rule below that, just as time does on the stones in strongman. So, anyone who closes a CoC No. 3 beats anyone who only closes a CoC No. 2, for example, but 14 reps on a CoC No. 2 beats 12 reps on the No. 2.

"The whole concept of 'ASC Live' is to reach out to the American fan base," Dione Wessels said. "What better way . . . than with the IronMind Grip Challenge?

The IronMind Grip Challenges will be taking place in at least six events across the country."

Incidentally, don't think you have to be a man to compete in these contests: "I have a stronger grip than a lot of guys," said Dione Wessels, who won the women's class at the 2003 U.S. Rolling Thunder National Championships, held in conjunction with Jim Davis's 2003 X-treme Strongman American Championships. M

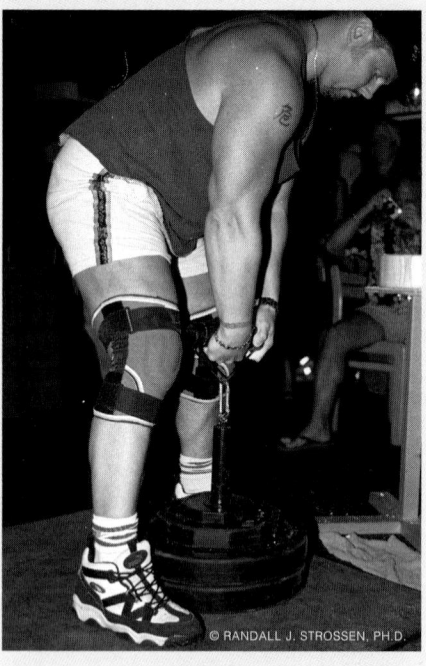

That's four-time World's Strongest Man winner Magnus Ver Magnusson getting ready to pull, just to give you an idea of the talent pool at some of the Rolling Thunder contests.
Randall J. Strossen photo.

Who's New

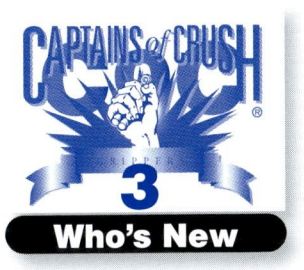

These two dynamos closed the No. 3 Captains of Crush Gripper* and have been added to the certified list:

Brad Ardrey
Rich Williams
Sam Solomi

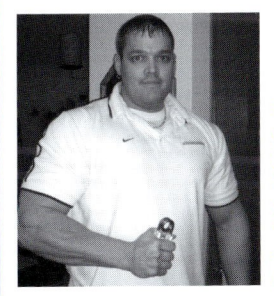

Brad Ardrey convinced judge Wade Gillingham on the No. 3 "no problem" at the 2009 Arnold.

Brad Ardrey, of Lancaster, Ohio, is 27 years old, 285 lb., and 6' 2" tall. Married to "my wonderful wife Angie, we just had a baby girl," Lyla, in September 2008. Brad is a salesman for U.S. Structures, and has been lifting weights for 10 years and competing in strongman for 6: "I train with Team B.O.S.S. (Brothers Of Stone & Steel) out of Columbus . . . we train 5 events (with one grip event) every Saturday morning starting at 6:30 a.m., and my favorite is the Atlas Stones." Brad hopes to officially close the No. 3.5 CoC at next year's Arnold . . . and to turn pro in strongman "and be on World's Strongest Man some day." Brad's come close to going pro "so maybe 2009 is my year." We wish you success, Brad!

Rich Williams made history by closing the No. 3 and the No. 3.5 Captains of Crush Grippers on the same day at the 2009 Arnold Sports Festival. The first person to double-certify, Rich's story is on page 75.

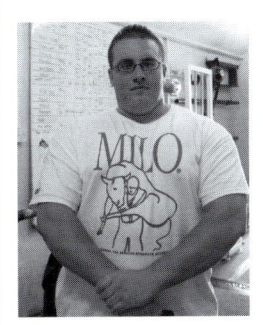

Sam Solomi "made it look so easy, closing it using his left hand for the cert and then just for fun with his right hand with a bit more effort!" noted witness Brian Phillips.
Brian Phillips photo.

Sam Solomi hails from Torbay, southwest England; he is 19 years old, 5' 8" and 280 lb.

Sam has not only certified on the benchmark No. 3 Captains of Crush Gripper, but as a mere 19-year old, he met the Jesse Marunde First Teenage Captains of Crush Gripper Challenge— the first to do so—and his tremendous accomplishment means that IronMind® is contributing US$500 to the educational fund for Jesse Marunde's children.

Sam co-owns a strongman gym "where we have just one rule which is TRAIN HARD." His best achievements in grip training include lifting a Thomas Inch DB replica and pulling over 100-kg on

*For a complete list of those certified on the No. 3, No. 3.5, and No. 4 Captains of Crush Grippers, or for the Rules for Closing and Certification, please visit the IronMind website at www.ironmind.com.

a Rolling Thunder. Sam says, "My first love is grippers; I have nearly 40 in total, including 8 different No. 3s! I hope to eventually certify on the No. 3.5 and . . . the No. 4." Sam has another goal, "to squat 180 kg for 20 reps. I have been motivated to do this after seeing Jesse Marunde's video of this feat. I did 10 reps recently so I think this is achievable." Sam works night shifts in a petrol station, "but I recently qualified as a personal trainer so hopefully I will be able to combine work and training and be one of the few people who earn money doing what they love!" We know you can do it, Sam! **M**

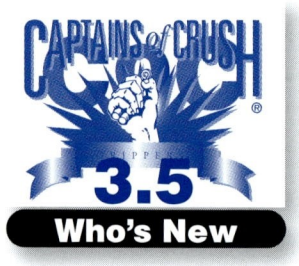

Who's New

Congratulations to these grip stalwarts for closing the No. 3.5 Captains of Crush Gripper:

Gabriel Sum
Rich Williams

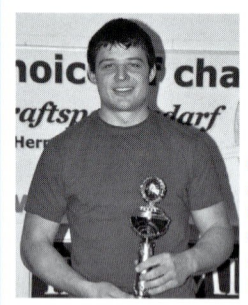

Gabriel Sum and his trophy from the 2009 Grip Nationals.
Courtesy of Dr. Hermann Korte.

Just about a year ago Gabriel Sum, of Troningen, Germany, was certified for closing the No. 3 Captains of Crush Gripper, and the young man whom Hermann Korte calls "just an amazing guy" has done it again, this time on the No. 3.5. At 1.83 m (6'-0"), 21 years old and 96 kg (212 lb.), Gabriel won the 2009 Grip Nationals for the second time, winning all four events and setting a German record on the Apollon's Axle with 172.5 kg; he also pinch gripped 110 kg with both hands. Gabriel came in second in last year's European Championships, which Dr. Korte also organized at his Choice of Champions Gym in Haltern. You're going strong, Gabriel! **M**

The first to do this, Rich Williams of Columbia, South Carolina, has certified on both the No. 3 and the No. 3.5 Captains of Crush Grippers at the same time. Rich is 30 years old and one of the big boys, weighing in at 395 lb. at 6' 3". Not surprisingly, he played football at Gardner-Webb University and was a three-time All-American. Married, with two children, Rich works fulltime with Team-Impact Ministries, traveling in the U.S. and throughout the world doing feats of strength and preaching the Gospel of Jesus Christ. Rich says, "I love to powerlift and do strongman training. My best lifts are 800-lb. raw deadlift, just a belt; 605 raw bench; 800 raw squat; 435 overhead axle press and 511 double overhand axle deadlift; 247 each hand on the new Rolling Thunder; upright row with the 202-lb. Circus Dumbbell; and 545 incline press. Rich trains at Sorinex with Richard and Bert Sorin: "I love being around people who love to train, not train to live." Of gripmaster Richard Sorin, he says: "In my book he is one of the best." Two thumbs up, Rich. What's next? **M**

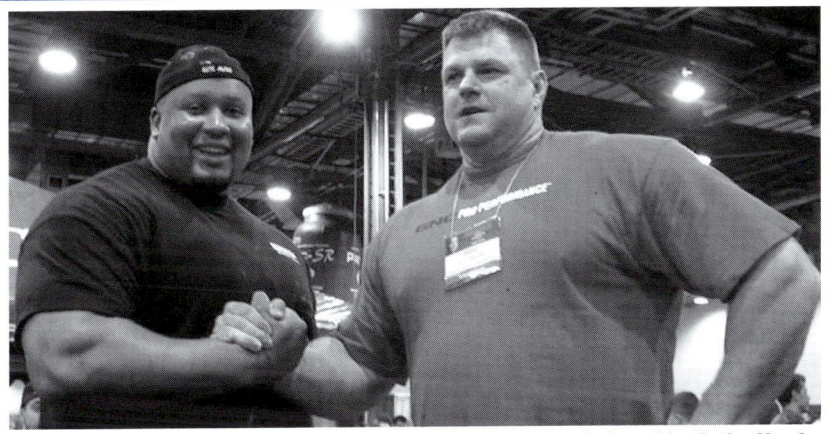

Rich Williams (l.) stopped by the GNC Grip Gauntlet and closed both the No. 3 and the No. 3.5 Captains of Crush Grippers on the same day at the 2009 Arnold Sports Festival where Wade Gillingham was our official on-site witness for the weekend. Here, Rich gets a congratulatory handshake from Brad Gillingham (r.).
Photo courtesy of Richard Sorin.

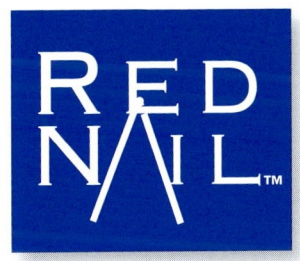

Red Nail™

R O S T E R

Four steel-fingered guys have mastered this short-steel bending feat and earned a place on the Red Nail Roster:

Derek Graybill
Henrik Nystrom
Jim Ricchezza
Mike Krahling

For a complete list of the Red Nail Roster or for the Rules and Certification for Bending a Red Nail, please visit the IronMind website at
www.ironmind.com.

Derek Graybill of Tucson, Arizona, is a mere youth at 16, standing 5' 11" and weighing 168 lb. He's competed in several grip contests in the area and participated in group training sessions put on by Red Nail-certified Aaron Corcorran, who has graciously served as an IronMind witness on several occasions. Derek has been lifting for 2-1/2 years and training his grip for only 18 months: "I've come a long way . . . I began very skinny and bending a white nail." Derek has also lifted the Blob plus 7.7 lb. (his PR) and hopes to certify on the No. 3 CoC before turning 17: "I hope to achieve a lot of great things because I started so early." You've got a good head start, Derek! M

Derek Graybill folded his Red Nail in just under 13 seconds and gets a congratulatory handshake from witness Aaron Corcorran.
Courtesy of Aaron Corcorran.

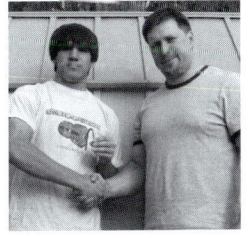

Henrik Nystrom has a deadly combination of persistence and patience.
Courtesy of Henrik Nystrom.

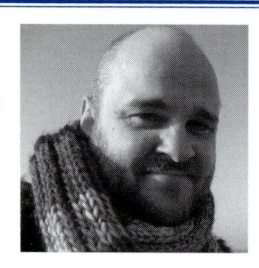

Henrik Nystrom of Gothenburg, Sweden, had to return to "Go" when his first-attempt Red Nail was lost in the mail but, persistent guy that he is, he redid the feat without missing a beat and his patience paid off with success. At 35 years old and 1.81 m (5' 11"), Henrik started bending about a year ago after seeing Red Nail-certified Brett Jones on YouTube and thinking, "That looks kind of cool." At first Henrik struggled with the white nails: "I spent my childhood and teens playing the piano and violin . . . it doesn't make your hands strong so I really had to start from the very beginning." See what we mean about persistence! Henrik has done some powerlifting but prefers old-school strongman-type training. The legend is that one of his ancestors built a barn all by himself with only an axe as a tool "so perhaps it is in my genes." We're sure of it, Henrik! **M**

Jim Ricchezza of Cherry Hill, New Jersey, liked the IronMind Hand Pads that he ordered shortly before he went for his Red Nail certification and wants to continue training with them: "They provide much more of a challenge and will definitely make you a stronger steel-bender." Having done a 6" Red Nail, Jim plans on going shorter . . . and then moving on to the Captains of Crush Grippers "to see how far I can go with them."

Jim also held the number-two place in the world in braced bending with 5/8" steel at 23-1/2" in length "but was recently bumped while training for my Red Nail cert." Jim is 33 years old, 5' 10" and 205 lb. Congrats, Jim—keep up the good work!

Mike Krahling of Exton, Pennsylvania, asked if he could tag along with Jim Ricchezza and go for his Red Nail certification at the same time. Mike, who is 38 years old, 6' 0" and 280 lb., started bending only 5 months ago! He has been training with kettlebells for the past 2-1/2 years under the guidance of Brian Petty RKC and attributes his bending progress to "the hand and upper-body strength I have gained from using kettlebells and the coaching by Jim Ricchezza in the proper form of bending." Mike and Jim did their bends at Steve Pulcinella's Iron Sport Gym in Glenolden, Pennsylvania, under the watchful eye of attorney Sean Burke, the official judge, who noted about each bend, "It was very well done." Way to go, Mike! **M**

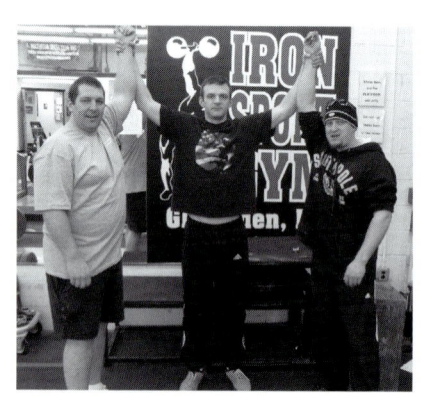

The winners! Jim Ricchezza (r.) and Mike Krahling (l.) flank official judge Sean Burke after their successful bends at Iron Sport Gym.
Steve Pulcinella photo.

2009 Arnold Arm Wrestling Challenge:
Tough Matches at the Top Tournament

Denise Wattles
Executive Director, United States Armwrestling

Twenty-five years ago United States Armwrestling held its first tournament in a small bar in Billings, Montana. Almost twenty-five years later to the day, we found ourselves (for the sixth time) on the main stage at the Arnold Sports Festival, showcasing our sport in front of thousands of spectators. The Arnold fitness expo includes dozens of sports, like bodybuilding, weightlifting, and strongman competitions, and recently MMA cage fighting, but of greatest importance to us is the most prestigious armwrestling event in the world, the Arnold Classic Armwrestling Challenge (ACAC).

Five countries were represented in the armwrestling competition this year. World champions Vazgen Soghoyan (Armenia) and Roman Tsindeliani (Russia) faced each other in the 154-lb. class. For the first time Poland sent not one but four of their top athletes to participate. Yes, armwrestling has evolved into a sport with some of the most talented and dedicated athletes in the world, but it also includes the "weekend warriors" who attend the many smaller events that the USAA holds nationwide.

Bill Logsdon has been competing for several years, and I had considered him one of the "weekend warriors"—until this weekend. The right-hand 177–198-lb. division at the ACAC has always been one of the toughest to place in. For the first time that I can remember there was not a current or previous ACAC champion in the class. Defending ACAC champion Michael Selearis was home awaiting the arrival of his first child, so this year someone new would have the thrill of winning the Arnold for the very first time. I have to say that Brent Rakers was favored to take home the title; and Mariusz Grochowski of Poland, in his first appearance at the Arnold, was an unknown to all of us and a "wild card" in how this class would shake out.

Defeating Byron Royer right out of the gate, Bill Logsdon exuded determination. Steve Rau beat Jeff Penney (Canada), last year's fourth-place finisher, in the first round and then handed Brent Rakers his first loss in the second. The physiques of Bill Logsdon and Steve Rau could not be more different. Bill is tall and lanky while Steve is compact and very muscular.

One can only assume based on appearance that Bill wouldn't have a chance against the more menacing Steve. At the Arnold the elimination rounds are held on Friday with the finals on Saturday. When Bill and Steve met in the semifinal match, Bill literally flashed Steve on the "Go," pounding him to the pad for a loss.

> ONE CAN ONLY ASSUME BASED ON APPEARANCE THAT BILL WOULDN'T HAVE A CHANCE AGAINST THE MORE MENACING STEVE.

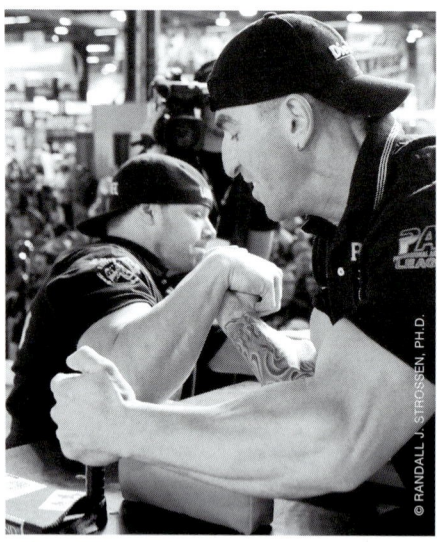

Steve "Razor" Rau (r.) had Bill Logsdon's (l.) number, but Bill's performance boosted his stock to a new level.
Randall J. Strossen photo.

At the end of the elimination rounds, it was Bill Logsdon who remained on the A-side undefeated, with Brent Rakers and Steve Rau on the B-side shaking their heads and re-thinking what move would put them back in the running. On Saturday, Steve "Razor" Rau must have replayed the previous day's match enough times to figure out how to beat Bill. Steve took home the ACAC title, beating Bill twice in the finals. Brent Rakers placed third and Mariusz Grochowski settled into the fourth place spot, happy with his finish in this stellar class.

This year's classes included three father-son and one father-daughter competitor combinations, proving that armwrestling is truly a family sport. Bill and Scott Ballinger, Gary and Jeremy Kessler, R. J. and Jay Molinere, and Todd and Sarah Opitz added a new twist to this event. The camaraderie and support of the parent-child relationships were absolutely inspiring.

Less than a week before the Arnold, the defending heavyweight champion, Richard Lupkes, was involved in a very serious auto accident in Minnesota, leaving him unable to attend. Previous ACAC champion Marcio Barboza (Brazil) was in Brazil for his wife's surgery and John Brzenk, two-time Arnold champion, had chosen to take a year off. The heavyweight title was up for grabs by any one of the men who had qualified to participate in this prestigious event. Tim Bresnan placed second last year so he definitely had the ability to finish in the top spot. Ron Bath had won the Arnold previously, but in 2006 and 2007 he placed "first after John." Ron's return this year, with John absent, might have been the time for him to regain the ACAC title. Michael Todd had attended the Arnold for the last four years but hadn't been able to place higher than second. Was

> THIS YEAR'S CLASSES INCLUDED THREE FATHER-SON AND ONE FATHER-DAUGHTER COMPETITOR COMBINATIONS, PROVING THAT ARMWRESTLING IS TRULY A FAMILY SPORT.

this the year for him to secure one of the most esteemed titles in the world?

Michael, looking strong from the start, dropped his opponents to the loser's bracket one by one until he ran into Ron Bath in the quarter finals. Ron had done the same, beating Dave Chaffee and Paul Fischer, before facing Michael Todd. Last year's second-place finisher, Tim Bresnan, fell to Michael Todd earlier in the bracket, making it harder on himself to work his way back to the finals. Tim suffered his second loss at the hand of Don "Hollywood" Underwood after several respectable wins on the B-side and finished out of the money. Mark Zalepa (Canada) definitely benefited from the luck of the draw. Drawing a bye in the first round set him up to place high in the bracket if he could pull out two consecutive wins.

In the past, Michael Todd has had a tough time with Ron Bath: Ron always competes at a high level and is normally successful in any event he attends but it seems he steps it up a notch when at the Arnold. Michael has given Ron some fierce matches at other events but when they meet at the Arnold, Ron's performance overshadows Michael's talent more than usual. I just don't get it, but that's how it was this year as well: Ron Bath regained the ACAC title, leaving Michael in second place, again. Mark Zalepa finished a very respectable third, with Don Underwood rounding out the top four.

Vazgen Soghoyan and Roman Tsindeliani, current world champions, gave defending champion R. J. Molinere all he could handle in the 154-lb. class. R. J. fell to Roman in the third round,

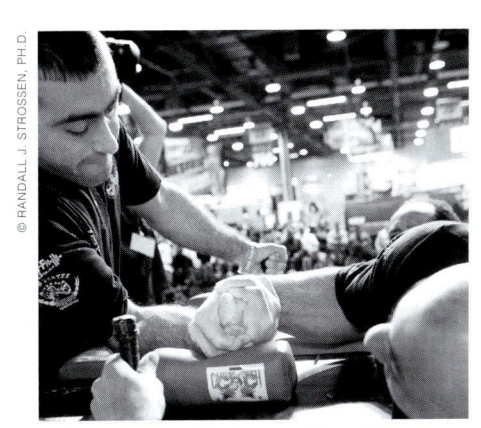

Both Vazgen Soghoyan (l.) and Roman Tsindeliani (r.) are world champions, but Roman smoked Vaz, providing a dominating response to whatever Vaz served up.
Randall J. Strossen photo.

reinforcing that it would be a tough battle to retain the Arnold title. Vazgen was also successful in dropping several top contenders to the loser's bracket quickly. Luke Kindt has been very successful lately in this class, but he had nothing for Vazgen.

Roman wrestled like a machine. Despite there being only about 10 pounds difference in their weight, when Vazgen and Roman met it was as though the battle was between a lightweight and heavyweight: Roman owned Vazgen. There was no move or technique that Vazgen could use to beat Roman. It was no surprise that Roman was crowned the 2009 154-lb. ACAC champion. Vazgen finished second, anticipating the opportunity to meet Roman again and have the chance to defeat him. R. J.'s only losses were to Roman and Vazgen, leaving him in third. Roger Nowatske, 2007 ACAC champion, rounded out the top four in this class.

> RON ALWAYS COMPETES AT A HIGH LEVEL AND IS NORMALLY SUCCESSFUL IN ANY EVENT HE ATTENDS BUT IT SEEMS HE STEPS IT UP A NOTCH WHEN AT THE ARNOLD.

One can't say enough about George Iszakouits (Canada). In spite of being 57 years old, George is one of the most feared armwrestlers in the 176-lb. class. George had an astounding record of holding six consecutive ACAC titles. He has defeated some of the biggest names in armwrestling, including Allen Fisher, Ron Klemba, Bill Ballinger, and the most challenging, James Smith. This weekend was no different. Herman McCoy has been able to tie up George for long matches in the past couple of years with his signature "dive," but drawing George in the first round may not have given Herman time to prepare mentally for his toughest opponent in this class. Herman lost to George in the first round and after beating Scott Ballinger on the B-side, he fell to Anthony Snook. George dominated all his matches, defeating Gary Kessler, Tomasz Szewszyk, and Andrew "Cobra" Rhodes before reaching the finals. Simon Berriochoa suffered a surprising loss to Justin Kopa in the second round, giving him a long path through the B-side to the possibility of prize money and maybe the coveted Arnold title.

Three wins later, Simon faced Cobra Rhodes in the battle for third place. In the past, Cobra had been tough for Simon to overcome, but Cobra was not on his game today. Hooking Cobra into his power, Simon came away the victor—but he still had infamously impregnable George Iszakouits in the finals. Simon placed higher than he ever has at the Arnold, but it was still second place to George. Seven consecutive titles will not make it easier for anyone to beat George next year! Cobra Rhodes and Tomasz Szewszyk placed third and fourth respectively.

The ladies' classes are lighter in attendance but they are always a crowd favorite. The stereotype that women armwrestlers resemble men more than women could not be further from actuality. The ladies who qualify for the

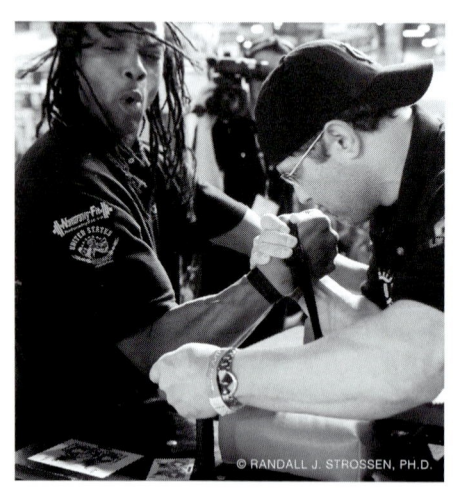

Cobra Rhodes (l.) looked like he was questioning the start, but it didn't matter because the power of Simon Berriochoa's (r.) hook was unstoppable.
Randall J. Strossen photo.

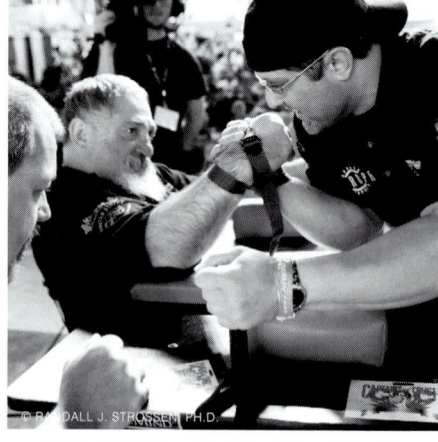

George Iszakouits (l.) settles into his favorite position against Simon Berriochoa (r.) in the finals: first George drops and then he wins.
Randall J. Strossen photo.

Arnold are very beautiful and also strong and skilled athletes. They, just like the men there, have had to qualify at a national, world, or international championships to participate in the Arnold Classic Armwrestling Challenge. Their matches are just as fierce and intense as any of the men's.

Tamara Mitts (Canada), in her sixth appearance since 2004, has won two ACAC titles. Margie Ciaccio is not only the defending champion but has at least three Arnold titles to her name. Placing behind Margie the last several years, Tamara has been training hard specifically to beat Margie at the Arnold. Tonya Todd has improved in leaps and bounds, and despite always giving up 10 to 20 pounds to the other ladies in this class, she proved her gains by placing third this weekend. Once again it was Margie and Tamara in the finals—and once again it was Margie who left Tamara in second place. The matches were still electrifying and still close, but the finish the same. Maybe 2010 will be Tamara's time.

> **NOT ONLY DID JOSEE COMPETE WITH A BROKEN LEG, SHE WON!**

In the third year of the ladies 144–176-lb. division, Josee Morneau (Canada) competed despite breaking her leg during a World's Strongest Woman competition two weeks earlier. Joyce King (who sponsors the prize money in this class) was unable to attend due to family commitments but was definitely there in spirit. Not only did Josee compete with a broken leg, she won! Finishing second was Darlene Ingledue, with Sarah Opitz taking third place.

The Arnold Classic Armwrestling Challenge would not be possible without the sponsorship and support of Iron Mind and Captains of Crush® Grippers. Randall and Elizabeth help us year-round and are true believers in our sport. They are both greatly appreciated! For the last six years, Fairfax Hackley had been the "wind beneath the wings" of armwrestling at the Arnold. Hack is a wonderful friend and a big advocate for us. Thanks so much, Hack! We also want to express our appreciation to Eric Hillman of Europa Sports for its sponsorship for the last two years. It is a huge help with the expenses for this event, including the thousands awarded in prize money. Last, but not least, thanks to Tony Nowak for donating the custom Arnold jackets presented to the winners in each division each year. The champions wear them with pride year-round. ∎

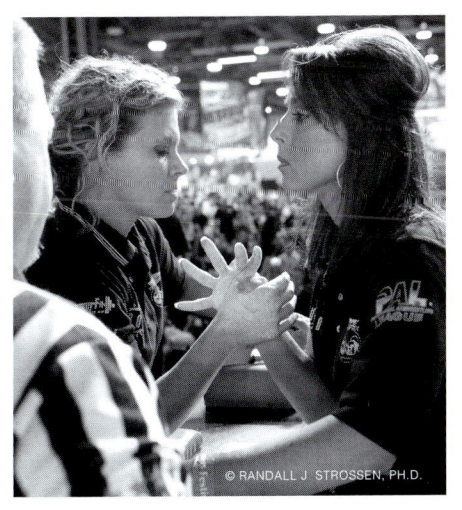

Tamara Mitts (l.) and Tonya Todd (r.) square off, ready to dispel stereotypes about what women armwrestlers look like and how hard they can pull.
Randall J. Strossen photo.

Building a High School Weightlifting Program
Success at Sac High

Paul Doherty

Coach, Sacramento High School

Coaches all across the U.S. can attest to the truly daunting and demanding task of building a weightlifting program at any level, and the incredible effort it requires. In this article, I'd like to focus on where that labor is concentrated rather than on the obvious amount of work it takes to build national championships-caliber athletes and teams.

We at Hassle Free have been fortunate to have had some success winning multiple national team championships at the School-Age and Junior Nationals. Furthermore, we have enjoyed considerable success with individual kids who have won national titles and earned spots on both Pan American and World teams. The observations that follow are based primarily on the successes and shortcomings of our club and may not represent a blueprint for future clubs. Our hope is, however, that others can learn from our mistakes as well as improve on our strong points. With that said, I generally get most of the credit for the program we have developed here in Sacramento, but I wanted to be sure and recognize Dave Swanson and Kari Shimomura, who volunteer their time and talents and really make our program go. Without them, our weightlifting program would not produce the quantity or quality of athletes that we do.

Recruit to win

The best athletes in the world walk the streets of our cities, and more specifically the hallways of our schools, every day and wait impatiently for someone to latch on to their talent and open the doors to bigger stages and arenas where they can flourish and flaunt their powers. The physical specimens we all drink in on Sundays (we're talking football, for you real dorks out there) are without a doubt among the elite athletes on the planet. Their physical talents and gifts mirror and complement snatching and clean and jerking so perfectly that an impeccable triple extension is waiting to tie itself around a bar and hoist it overhead for world-record lifts.

Yet, we've lost before we've started. We have high standards and expect these athletes to want to lift on their own without ever being exposed to the fascination we all share for the sport. We can't hope and wait for the iron bug to bite them. We literally have to strap them to a gurney and pour a bucketful of famished iron bugs on them and let the bugs feast. I exaggerate for effect here because too frequently coaches become discouraged by athletes who don't share their passion. This is normal! Before being exposed to weightlifting at the dreadfully-late age of 18, I used to love basketball more than any other sport.

You first have to expose them, and then, if you're really single-minded as my brother Kevin and I are, you give them no choice but to participate. You force them to go to training sessions and meets and eliminate every possible excuse for them not to be able to go. You hunt them down on the street corner after school and drag them to the squat rack. You pick them up from the bus stop and lock them in the weight room. Saturday morning you pull them up out of bed and throw them in the trunk of your car on your way to a meet. You brainwash them into a dazed and confused state, baffled at how they could possibly think weightlifting was "uncool." And you do this by showing your own enthusiasm. You do it all with a smile on your face, overflowing fervor, and a reckless agenda to promote the sport. You live and eat the sport and breathe that life into those athletes. You have to make it happen. They don't wake up and choose weightlifting on their own. Ninety-nine percent of our (Kevin and my) energy, as silly as it may seem and as critical as people may be of it, is spent on actively chasing down kids on campus and bringing them with us to the weight room. Over time, the kids start to hunt each other down; they police themselves and are perplexed at the very notion of going anywhere else but the platform after school.

We must protect and nurture their fragile egos, but at the same time push them to new heights of accomplishment. I am absolutely convinced beyond any shadow of doubt that these same athletes you see on TV day in and day out would choose weightlifting—just the same as they would football or basketball—if only they had familiarity with the sport. I only wish that every iron fan out there who lives and breathes snatches and clean and jerks would walk into their neighborhood high school every day and pluck these athletes right off the tree and watch them ripen on the platform and bloom into spectacular lifters. The high school halls and lunchtime commons are where the world-class athletes wait. Even better, the middle schools and junior highs they come from have plenty of willing stars and future champions. Too often gym rats paint themselves into a corner by starting gyms or working at health clubs that attract no one in the right age group to win the Olympics. We have to be in schools and start programs on campuses to really develop athletes at the ripe early age of 10 to 14 years.

> YOU HUNT THEM DOWN ON THE STREET CORNER AFTER SCHOOL AND DRAG THEM TO THE SQUAT RACK.

Build a monopoly

Fantastic! Now that your brilliant coaching efforts are focused on the right age group in the right school district, work harmoniously with your colleagues to help build the program that should be found on every high school campus. We have been tremendously blessed at Sacramento High to have the full support of the administration for our weightlifting programs. School administration and leaders like P. K. Diffenbaugh, Herinder Pagany, Jim Scheible, Ed Manasala, and Kevin Johnson all contribute by promoting, supporting and allowing our program to flourish.

Too often have I read in publications or overheard in conversations about football being the arch enemy of weightlifting—and far too frequently do I hear about schemes and strategies in

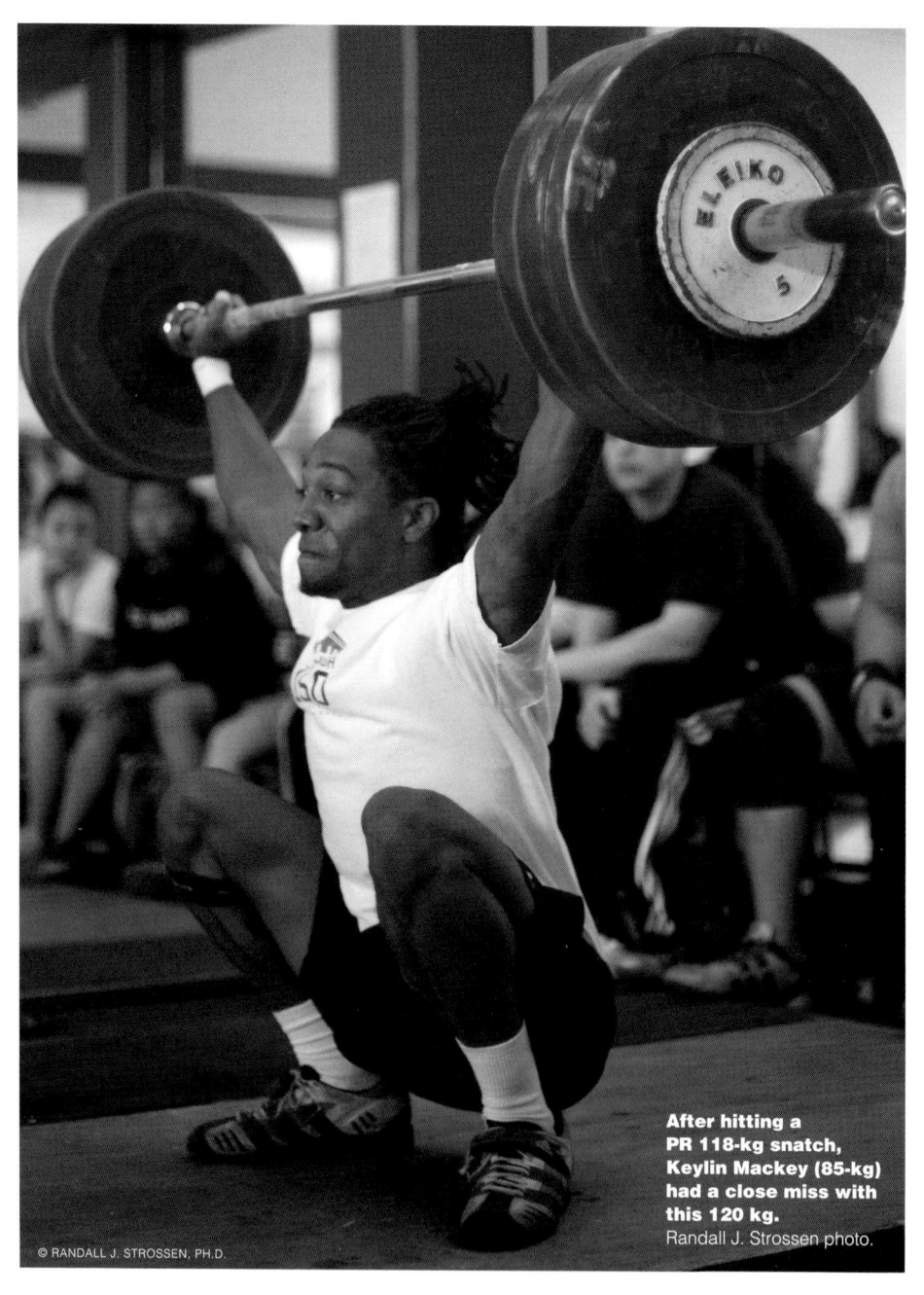

After hitting a PR 118-kg snatch, Keylin Mackey (85-kg) had a close miss with this 120 kg.
Randall J. Strossen photo.

motion to dissuade athletes from pursuing gridiron glories. Frankly, all sports are necessary for the general preparation of athletes in our sport, and they serve their purpose.

Do yourself a favor—COACH FOOTBALL! What better recruiting tool could you possibly conceive? At Lincoln High School in San Francisco (winners of five straight section championships), Kevin Doherty cut 17 returning varsity players form his roster in 2003 when they couldn't clean 100 kg. I don't give a running back the ball unless he's on the weightlifting team. Don't believe me? Keylin Mackey, who won the silver medal at this year's Junior Nationals and missed out on a Junior World spot by a hair, started as a running back before Clinton Johnson, the fifth-place finisher in the clean and jerks of that same session at the Nationals, took over after Keylin graduated.

> DO YOURSELF A FAVOR—COACH FOOTBALL! WHAT BETTER RECRUITING TOOL COULD YOU POSSIBLY CONCEIVE?

My brother makes weightlifting meets mandatory football practice. It's annoying and stressful to some hosts who'd rather not see a hundred-plus 20-and-under lifters at their events on a Saturday, but it's necessary for our club to generate the numbers we do.

Strength in numbers

Our club's approach from the very beginning was to put a priority on the School-Age Nationals (and move on up the ranks from there) in order to push as many athletes as possible through the funnel while experiencing as much success as possible. Furthermore, the emphasis has *always* been on team success as opposed to individual accomplishment. Clearly weightlifting is an individual sport that celebrates the accomplishments of the sole athlete atop the podium; however, getting there certainly is easier when you expand (exponentially at times) the pool of athletes plugged into the pipeline. Coincidentally, this approach pays off in more ways than one at initial glance. Let me explain.

I spent three weeks in Fuzhou, China during the summer of 2007. This training center serves as home to athletes such as Zhang Jie and Lu Chang Liang. Both, conveniently, won the Asian Games in 2008 after making appearances at the IronMind Invitational at the Arnold Classic in March. This training center is one of the best in the whole country and boasts world-record lifts daily that I can personally attest to. But it is still one of 30 just like it throughout the country. They had upward of 40 platforms and approximately 90 world-class lifters. I will not spend much time on their training program as it is well-documented and is perhaps material for another article, but I will comment on the sheer number of top-level lifts I saw day in and day out.

Perhaps the best example of this was the 184-kg clean and jerk on a Wednesday morning by Jie, winner of the 2008 Asian Championships in the 62-kg class. Dumbfounded first at the ridiculous strength, agility, and athleticism of the act as I stood 10 feet away, I was more in shock that he was not even on the national team roster! His explanation: "Snatch is too far behind. Only 147." It's true that some top lifts

> ... I WAS MORE IN SHOCK THAT HE WAS NOT EVEN ON THE NATIONAL TEAM ROSTER! HIS EXPLANATION: "SNATCH IS TOO FAR BEHIND. ONLY 147."

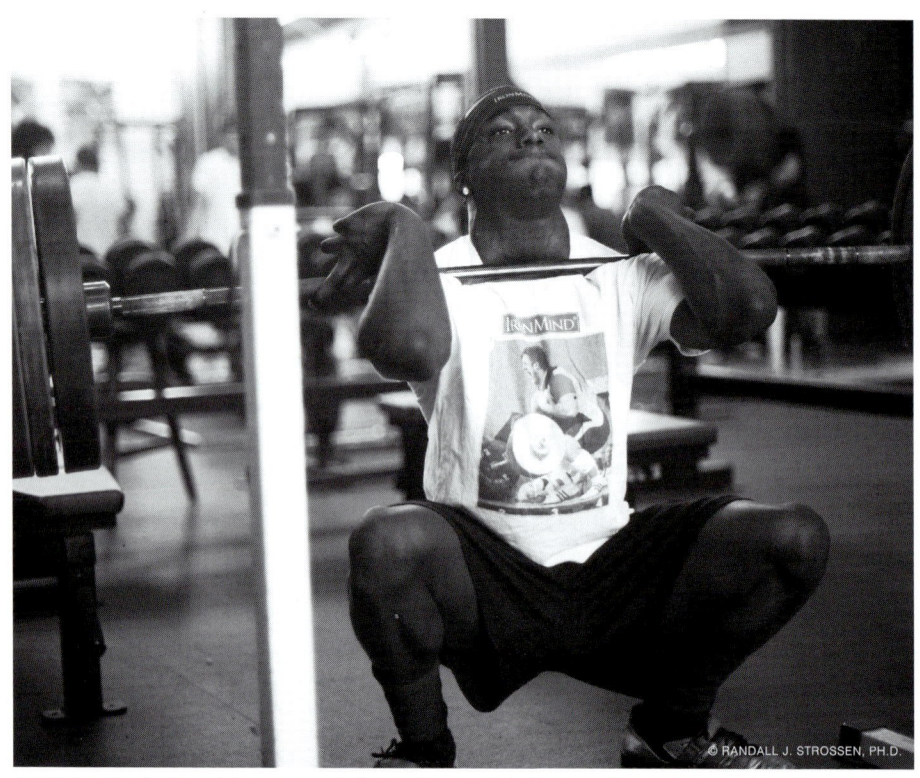

2009 Junior National bronze medalist in the snatch, Byron Gibson has outstanding athletic ability, cleaning and jerking what he front squats!

Paul Doherty notes: "Byron is a perfect example of what our program is all about. Byron started as a struggling junior in high school facing tough academic and social obstacles, but has been on an upward climb since then. Just 19, he has been supporting himself, working full-time and going to school while training. I view Byron as our most mature and developed lifter, handling real life comfortably and on his way to a long weightlifting career.

"Byron is close to, if not the, most athletic lifter we have. He cleans and jerks what he front squats, caught touchdown passes with ease, and can jam a basketball by just touching it. When his bodyweight and strength catch up to his athleticism, he will be atop the podium. Byron's best lifts as a 77 are 110 and 130. Byron won a bronze medal in the snatch in the 77-kg weight class at the Junior Nationals this year, snatching what he cleaned and jerked just a year ago. This will be the last time you see him in the 77s: he will be skipping the 85s and moving straight to the 94s hopefully by May."

Randall J. Strossen photo.

but nowhere would you find a total that surpassed his in 2008. He went on to clean and jerk 179 kg at the Asian Championships and total 326 kg, with that 147-kg snatch. The winning total at the Olympics? The 319 kg by China's Zhang Xiangxiang.

After seeing this, I thought back to our broken conversation the year before and recalled the reason for his absence on the roster: "Snatch is too far behind." Perhaps most unbelievable was that everyone in the room, from his friends, coach, and training partners

69-kg Kyle Saelee broke his wrist when he missed a 135-kg clean, but he never missed a day of training and that didn't stop him from attacking this 190-kg squat, no wraps and no spotters. Randall J. Strossen photo.

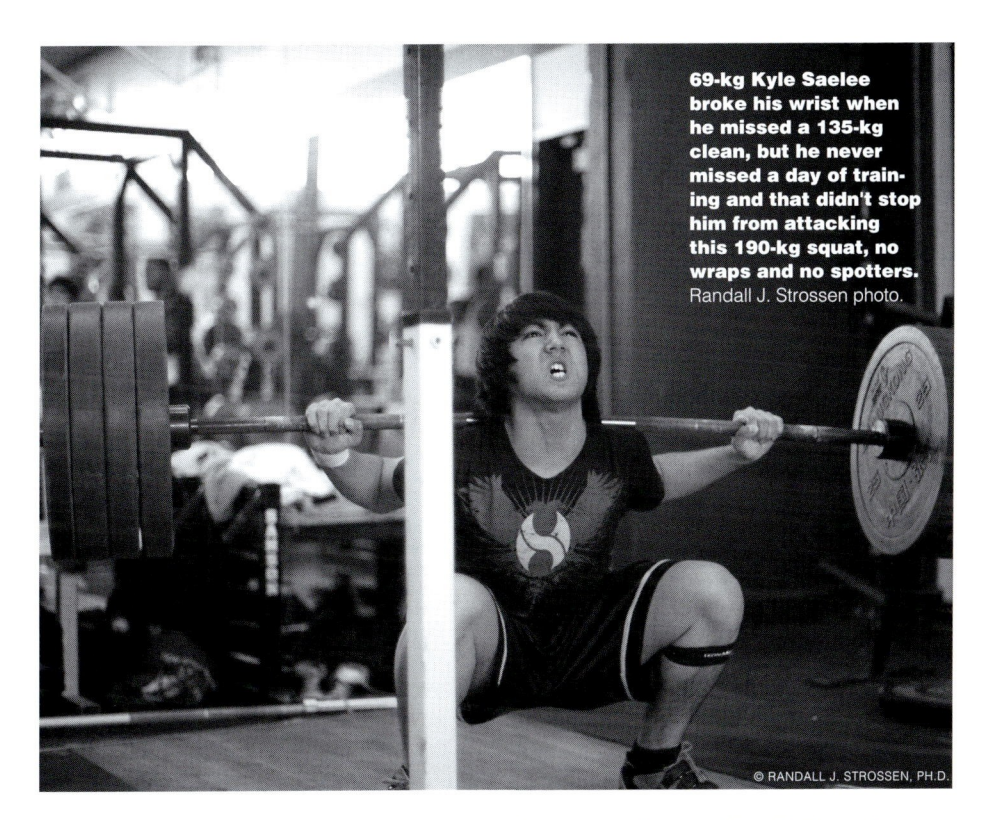

to the cooks and janitors, was in agreement. China couldn't afford to put an athlete on stage that would have to play catch-up. They all took it as normal and resigned themselves to the most basic response any highly-educated coach could possibly fathom, "train harder," in the most matter-of-fact manner you could find.

Clearly one can comprehend the value of having strength in numbers for a team to have their pick of any medal they choose at any given contest, but at our grassroots level it plays a different role. It's true; we frequently have multiple athletes in Junior National Championships on the medal stand. For example, in the 56-kg class at this year's Juniors, we had Sae Vang and Chris Tiongson winning the silver and bronze medals respectively, as well as Keylin Mackey and Ian Wilson doing the same in the 85-kg class. But what you might not know is that we also had Harold Davis and Clinton Johnson—who were not in medal contention—competing in those sessions. These are two athletes from whom we expect future success at the Junior Nationals and beyond, and bringing them helps their overall development as they gain experience.

However, more so they are two extra bodies in the stands supporting their teammate Donavan Ford when he goes for a personal-record clean and jerk of 180 kg. It is two more mouths on campus pushing the weightlifting agenda and spreading the clean and jerk propaganda. It creates a fan base, adds to the pre-contest hype, and helps promote my soapbox speeches that drone on

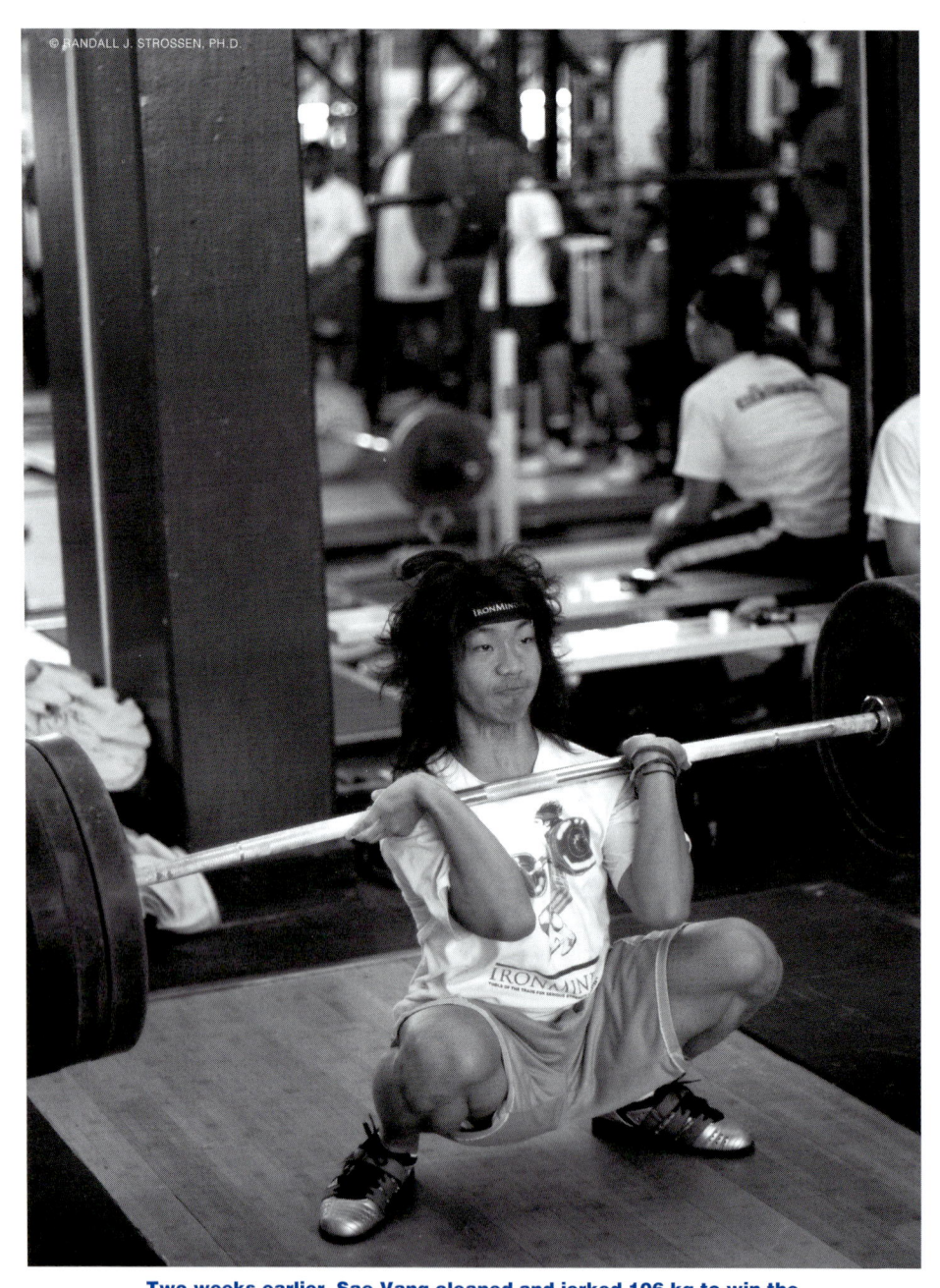

Two weeks earlier, Sae Vang cleaned and jerked 106 kg to win the Junior Nationals. The day Randall Strossen visited Sac High, Sae Vang cleaned and jerked 107 kg for a PR. Next, although he was nearly buried by the weight, Sae Vang managed to clean this 110 kg and he gave jerk a good shot. Everyone who has seen him lift has two words to say about Sae Vang: watch out! Some background on Sae Vang from coach Paul Doherty: "Sae Vang is one of 11 kids living in a two-bedroom house in Oak Park. He never complains, shows up every day, and just kicks butt. Watch out for him!"

Randall J. Strossen photo.

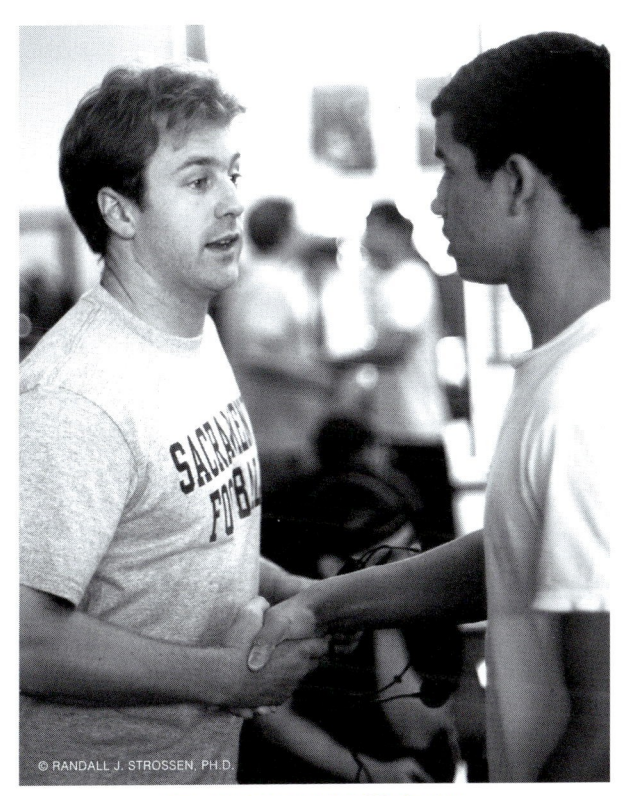

**Sac High coach Paul Doherty:
"Making a difference, not a dollar."**
Randall J. Strossen photo.

for hours at a time throughout the duration of a training session. Denis Reno said it best when our team took the platform at the 2008 Junior Nationals to receive the first-place team award: "If they all come up to receive the trophy . . . there goes our audience." Everyone had a laugh at his comment, but it was true. We had 23 of the 110 athletes on the start list and 27 more bussed down by the school (and principal) on that last day to share in the celebration. *To share in the celebration.* They all celebrated because they were a part of the winning team, even though only a few of our athletes scored points to contribute to the win. But that's not what I tell them. I tell them that each and every lift they make is scored and that they are just as much responsible for the team win as Sae Vang's 106-kg gold-medal clean and jerk.

All of these athletes cannot win the Olympics, but they create a community within which a future Olympic champion can thrive. The program is now literally bigger than the athlete. Helping out at this year's Juniors was one of my very first lifters, Brian Hurwick, who had a third-place finish at the 2006 School-Age Nationals and earned himself a spot on the 17-under Pan Am team that competed in Venezuela later that fall. He was there with his other teammate, David Garcia, who won silver in the snatch at that contest and was expected to make the Junior World roster this year before having shoulder surgery. Both of them helped load, coach, and cheer. After high school I knew it was highly unlikely that Brian would continue lifting, but I pushed him through the funnel anyway, and now, as a 20-year-old college student, he flew home from Denver just to help load and break down the meet.

As any meet director can attest to, it takes a full crew to run these events and many hands make for light work. The 50 or so young, able bodies that were representing Hassle Free at the 2009 Junior Nationals all broke down a stage and competition platform that boasted 140 sheets of plywood in less than a half hour, a task that took the meet organizers over four hours to set up prior to the meet. When they all got back to the campus after the weekend, not only were there 23 athletes talking about the overwhelming success of the contest, but 27 of their teammates as well. Fifty mouths were talking to 100 ears about weightlifting, and the buzz grows and recruits yet another young lifter to the funnel.

Create the culture

Now you've created a whole culture. Campus life is booming with weightlifters. Better yet, if you happen to land in one of my three weightlifting classes that each holds 75 students on 25 platforms every day, you hear it constantly. That's 225 kids out of 1,000 in a school for whom weightlifting is now even more normal than the NFL network. My propaganda drowns out *SportsCenter*, and snatches are as familiar to them as jump shots. This doesn't include the hundreds (literally) more who train before and after school.

Expectations

Tommy Kono says it best: "Expect to win the international medals as much as the national medals and you will. Shoot higher. Aim for Olympic gold rather than the Olympic team." I took this to heart when I first started at Sacramento High and thought it would take years for me to duplicate the success my brother was enjoying in San Francisco. But I set the bar high: international medal in the first year. And guess what, the kids don't know any different. I latched on to a few

> TOMMY KONO
> SAYS IT BEST:
> ..."AIM FOR
> OLYMPIC GOLD
> RATHER THAN THE
> OLYMPIC TEAM."

bunches of kids and set the normalcy of seven-days-a-week training. This kept them off the streets and in the weight room.

The Oak Park neighborhood, where most of my students come from, is swollen with poverty, hunger, societal diseases, and gang violence. Weightlifting was an escape for them. Training twice a day, five days a week and once on Saturday and Sunday was required. Guess what? They showed up. Why? Because I picked them up. Guess what happens when good athletes train really hard. Results. We finished that first year with three out of the five boys on the sub-15 Pan Am team: Chris Tiongson, Kyle Saelee, and Clinton Johnson. They only came home with a few medals, but were the number one team. Imagine that. They must have thought to themselves, crazy Coach Doherty was right again. I was shocked. They achieved more than I had expected and I was humbled by Tommy's words of wisdom.

Training environment

The one last element I'd like to discuss is the training environment. Showing up day in and day out—even on Christmas Day and Thanksgiving—at the same dusty weight room is a challenge and can wear on an athlete. There is no way they will progress without any new stimulus or catalyst to get them going. That's why they have each other. Most of the time their biggest competitor is training right next to them on the same platform every day. On three occasions we have had the

> THEY ARE CONSTANTLY REMINDED OF WHAT'S AT STAKE EVERY DAY WHEN THEY DRAG IN WITH AN EMPTY TANK, AND IT REFUELS THEM FOR VIGOROUS WORKOUTS.

ninth- or tenth-ranked boy for an international team behind two or three of his teammates who ranked fourth or fifth. The competition never ends. They are constantly reminded of what's at stake every day when they drag in with an empty tank, and it refuels them for vigorous workouts.

The first year I started (2006), I had four of the top-ten 15-under boys in the whole country in one P.E. class, and my brother had a fifth. The only reason they got there ahead of better weightlifters was because they had each other to train with. Two years later, during my same fifth-period weightlifting class, I have four of our best college lifters join them to take advantage of the dynamite training environment. Imagine a high school P.E. class with Donavan Ford, David Garcia, Keylin Mackey, Byron Gibson, Sae Vang, Brandell Sampson, Clinton Johnson, Kyle Saelee, Alex Lee and Trevon Johnson all training together. Better yet, imagine Casey Dudley and Harold Davis, two freshmen in the same class seeing this every day and having to keep up to earn a grade . . . and the ball just keeps on rolling. **M**

CALENDAR

Check out the Latest News at **www.ironmind.com**, the Strength World's News Source.

2009 NA Strongman, Inc.
For upcoming contest and information, visit www.nastrongmaninc.com or contact Willie and Dione Wessels, 314-770-9279, e-mail: dione@americanstrongman.com.

2009 United States Armwrestling Association, Inc.

Jun 6	1st Annual Black Hills Pro-Am AW Champs, Deadwood, SD
Jun 13	17th Annual Miller Kansas State AW Championship, Bonner Springs, KS
Jun 25-27	USAF Unified National AW Championships, Little Rock, AR
Jul 11	3rd Annual Oklahoma State Pro-Am AW Championship, Anadarko, OK
Jul 18	Mountain States Regional Armwrestling, Sterling, CO
Jul 25	Evel Knievel Days AW, Butte, MT
Jul 25	Nor-Cal State AW Champs, Redding, CA
Jul 25	North Dakota State AW Championship, Minot, ND
Jul 25	1st Annual Sturgis Bound Rally AW, Belen, NM
Aug 8	Wyoming State AW Championship, Douglas, WY
Aug 15	16th Annual Europa Super Show Pro-Am AW Challenge, Dallas, TX
Aug 22	Barley's Tournament of Champions Pro-Am AW, Hawthorne, NV
Aug 29	1st Annual Kentucky Showdown, Buckhorn, KY
Sep 6-12	WAF World AW Championship, Porto Viro, Italy
Oct 17	2009 Central Texas Showdown AW, Temple, TX
Nov 7	2009 Annual Great Falls Montana Open AW, Great Falls, MT

For more information, contact the USAA, 246 Custer Avenue, Billings, MT 59101; 406-248-4508 or 406-245-1560; www.usarmwrestling.com.

2009 United States All-Round W/L Assn.
For upcoming events and information, contact Bill Clark, 3906 Grace Ellen Drive, Columbia, MO 65202-1796. USAWA is a drug-free organization.

2009 Powerlifting
For scheduled events, check *Powerlifting USA* magazine. For subscription information, call 805-482-2378.

2009 USA Weightlifting/IWF

Jun 4-7	National & Pan Am Championships, Chicago, IL
Jun 12-21	Junior World Championships, Bucharest, Romania
Nov 17-27	World Championships, Goyang City, Korea
Dec 11-13	American Open, Mobile, AL

For more information on USA Weightlifting contests, please contact 719-866-4508 or www.usaweightlifting.org. For information about international competitions, please visit www.iwf.net.

2009 Highland Games
For schedules of competitions, please see the following websites:
. www.asgf.org
. www.saaa-net.org
. www.highlandnet.com
. www.nasgaweb.com

The Single-Hand Deadlift

Roger Davis

In his book *How to Use a Barbell* (1925 Edition), W. A. Pullum describes the deadlift and the right- and left-hand deadlift as "The fundamental tests of a man's bodily strength," and even with the advent of modern lifting equipment and training methods I believe that this still holds true.

The single-hand deadlift is one of the ultimate tests of a lifter's overall strength—the back and legs may be strong, but if the grip is weak, the bar remains on the floor and vice versa.

I will be including lifts performed on standard Olympic bars, cambered bars and unique lifting equipment, as well as introducing *MILO* readers to one of the most painful but effective methods of performing a heavy single-hand deadlift—the dreaded hook grip.

Before I provide you with the lifts that I have researched, it would be good for you to know the differences in using various pieces of equipment, so that you know we are comparing like-for-like lifts.

Equipment

Probably the easiest form of equipment to use for a single-hand deadlift is a raised weight, that is, a stone or block weight that puts the handle above the lifter's knee, with a round ring handle, which makes contact with more of the hand than a straight bar does. With such a set-up, the lifter does not require the same back strength as with a standard bar and plates, and the round shape of the handle helps. The Dinnie Stones have such a set-up although, as I can well testify, their sheer weight and awkwardness makes them more than a worthy challenge.

In Britain in the 1920s, W. A. Pullum developed a number of lifting bars specifically for the all-round weightlifter. One of these was the Pullum cambered bar, which was a shorter than usual barbell with a slight bend. Its advantage was that if the lifter positioned the bend slightly away from the palm, the bar would naturally turn into the hand and help considerably with the grip when lifting. Although I have never lifted on a cambered bar (they are collectors' items nowadays), some of my veteran lifting friends have recounted that such a bar had an effect very similar to a hook grip, and the bar locked itself into the palm. The majority of the British single-hand deadlifts prior to 1985 were performed on this equipment.

Interestingly, W. A. Pullum relates that when the mighty Hermann Goerner stayed with him for a visit, he enjoyed putting the camber into the bars. One can only imagine how the powerful Hermann did this—any way he liked, I guess!

A standard Olympic barbell gives us exactly what it says, a standard, and it is the easiest way to directly compare lifts. It is nice to see that the heaviest single-hand deadlift of all time was performed on a standard Olympic barbell; more on that later.

The fourth piece of equipment, and probably the most challenging on which any lift is performed, is a dumbbell or barbell that has a handle thicker than the usual 1", which has a significant, limiting effect on the grip.

Notable lifts

The first reported single-hand deadlifts that I can find come from the strongman era, and the standard of equipment cannot therefore be verified. Canadian strongman Arthur Dandurand is reported to have lifted 250 kg in a single-hand deadlift. His compatriot Louis Cyr lifted a 238-kg dumbbell with a 1.5" grip using one hand on 31 March 1896, a truly remarkable feat of grip strength and no doubt a result of Louis's continued training with thick-handled dumbbells.

August W. Johnson, the strongman from Sweden, is also reported to have lifted 215.5 kg single-handed at around 95-kg bodyweight in the late 1890s.

In his book *The Way to Live*, George Hackenschmidt recounts a visit to Munich in 1901 to the famed inn and weights room of the retired strongman Hans Steyrer. Among an assortment of stones and weights was a stone weighing 299.2 kg with a handle attached, which George proceeded to lift with one hand. There is no mention whether or not straps were involved with this lift; if not, it was a fantastic display of grip strength.

In Britain, Thomas Inch, using his grip made famous by his challenge dumbbell, performed a single-hand deadlift of 182.2 kg on a straight 1.25" barbell.

Somewhat later, weights and their specifications became more standardized so that we can now be sure of what is being described. The incomparable Hermann Goerner was the indisputable king of the single-hand deadlift on this standard equipment. On 29 October 1920 in Leipzig, Germany, he performed an officially-refereed 301 kg on the right-hand deadlift, although his unofficial record was a mind-blowing 330 kg performed just three weeks earlier at the same location on the same equipment.

This lift was performed on a Berg revolving barbell, and is a number that has never been approached and to my mind, like Arthur Saxon's bent press, never will be. It is interesting to note that Hermann performed his single-hand deadlifts with the bar in front of the body, rather than in the straddle position that was more favoured by British lifters.

Of his fellow continental lifters, Charles Rigoulot lifted 202.5 kg in Paris in 1926, and his arch rival Ernest Cadine just topped this with 204 kg, both very good lifts on the single-hand deadlift.

Records

The records on the single-arm deadlift for British lifters before World War II are as follows:

8 stone – J. A. Jenkins	149.7 kg (LH)*
9 stone – Arthur Hunt	165.8 kg (BH)
10 stone – Arthur Hunt	186.3 kg (BH)
12 stone – Laurence A. Chappell	227.6 kg (RH)
Heavyweight – Ronald Walker	199.9 kg (LH)

* RH = right hand, LH = left hand, BH = both hands

. . . HIS UNOFFICIAL RECORD WAS A MIND-BLOWING 330 KG . . .

There was a glut of record attempts on the single-hand deadlift in Britain in the mid-1930s, none more so than the numerous record attempts performed by the Hull weightlifter Arthur Hunt. Hunt broke the record on a number of occasions and claimed his 9-stone lifts as world records; it is very interesting to note that he managed to create the same record lifts with both his right and left hands—this is very unusual as most lifters favour one hand over the other.

In addition to weightlifting history, I also collect the memorabilia (especially medals and trophies) from this period and am actually the proud owner of a plaque presented to Arthur Hunt in recognition of his world-record lifts on the single-hand deadlift. This plaque was presented to Hunt by his good friend and fellow all-round weightlifter Ossie Knox, who at one time held the world record in the deadlift with a lift of 255.4 kg at 12 stone. Incidentally, Arthur Hunt was an undertaker by profession, and I have a number of anecdotes whereby he states that this is the reason that he was so good at the deadlift—his joke, not mine!

Laurence Chappell is also recorded as performing an unofficial single-hand deadlift of 253 kg at the very modest bodyweight of 75 kg—a truly remarkable feat that his mentor and coach, the professional strongman "Young Apollon" (J. C. Tolson), made a great deal of in his magazine advertisements for muscles by mail.

I do not have much information on American all-round lifters, but I have records of John Y. Smith lifting 204 kg with his right hand at the respectable age of 60 in 1926; heavyweight Malcolm Brenner performing a 250-kg single-hand deadlift in 1949; and heavyweight Steve Ekdal lifting 276.7 kg for a single and 181.3 kg for ten reps. The latter two individuals lifted with the bar to the front.

Peter B. Cortese of the U.S. completed a 168-kg single-hand deadlift in 1954 at the very modest bodyweight of 52.5 kg. In his book *Weight Lifting*, Bob Hoffman lists 104 kg, 122 kg and 143 kg as being first-class standards for light, middle and heavyweight lifters on the single-hand deadlift; these figures appear rather low to me.

I also have read that modern-day gripmaster Richard Sorin has lifted 226.7 kg on a barbell and 272 kg on a short-range movement with a lead-filled box with a 1.25" handle.

More up-to-date and on less-regular equipment, in 1983 the building block company Celcon ran a competition to see who could lift the most of their blocks with one hand—this was a partial lift on a suspended platform using a chain attached to the blocks and a D- or O-ring handle. The winner on this occasion was Clive Lloyd, who lifted a magnificent 303.5 kg; three months later, Willie Whoriskey broke this record with 304.3 kg.

Modern-day grip competitions on the short-range single-hand deadlift have produced lifts of 330 kg for Steve Gardner and 300 kg for David Horne—fantastic demonstrations of grip strength over a short range.

Although not listed as an IAWA world record as it was performed on a cambered bar, IAWA U.K. General Secretary and British all-round great Frank Allen performed an astonishing

230-kg right-hand deadlift at light heavyweight on 11 October 1981. This beat the record set by Laurence A. Chappell almost 50 years previous and was met with great delight.

Getting back to lifts performed on a standard Olympic barbell from the floor, some of the best lifts on the single-hand deadlift in modern competition are as follows:

	Kg	Bwt.
John McKean	147.5 kg (RH)*	60 kg
Steve Sherwood	200 kg (LH)	70 kg
Bob Hirsh	200 kg (LH)	80 kg
David Horne	220 kg (RH)	90 kg
Steve Angell	210 kg (LH)	100 kg
M. McBride	183.7 kg (RH)	110 kg
Frank Ciavattone	255.1 kg (RH)	120 kg

*RH = right hand; LH = left hand

As a guide, I would suggest that with continued progressive training a lifter really should be able to work up to 150% of his bodyweight on the single-hand deadlift, and more if employing a hook grip.

How to do the lift

To hook or not to hook, that is the question. If you are using the single-hand deadlift as a training tool to improve the grip, I would suggest that you do not hook and allow the grip to naturally develop its strength through progressive overload.

If, however, you are looking to complete a single-hand deadlift in competition (and unless you have a world-class grip far above your current back strength), I will say hook, hook, hook—you would be mad not to.

For illustration, my best unhooked single-hand deadlifts right- and left-handed are 130 kg and 120 kg, respectively. By

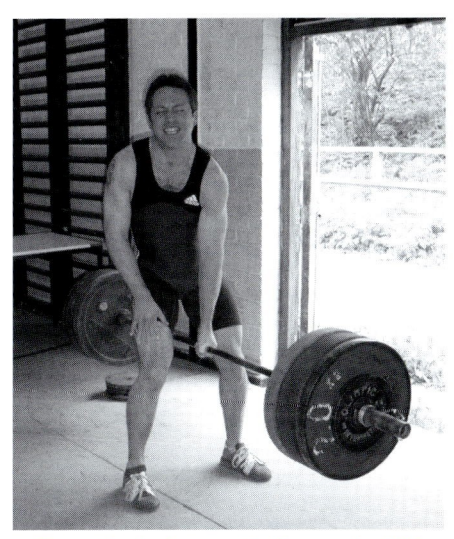

Roger Davis does a single-arm deadlift in competition.
Photo courtesy of Roger Davis.

applying a hook grip, they jump to 175 kg and 150 kg; that's roughly a 20–25% benefit to be had by hooking—a difference that you just cannot afford to give away in a competition.

I am sure that the majority of MILO lifters know how to apply a hook grip, but for those who don't, it is basically about wrapping the thumb as far under the bar as you possibly can and closing the remaining fingers over the thumb to hold it in position. When the bar is lifted, the thumb is locked into position and crushed between the bar and the fingers—very painful, but very effective.

Hook grip.

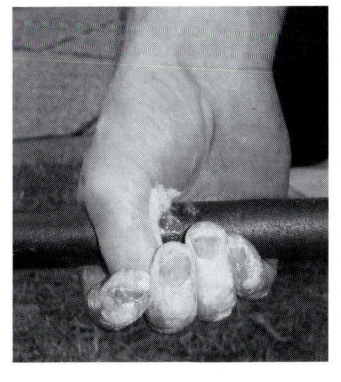

I find that an involuntary shout often helps the lifter get through the experience! You must be sure to continue squeezing the grip as tightly as possible, rather than just relying on the pressure on the thumb to hold the grip solid. A well-chalked hand and thumb can also help, and some lifters even go as far as using a small nail file to make the thumbnail more abrasive.

The next decision is whether to lift the bar in the traditional deadlift position or to straddle the bar—the choice is up to you, but in my opinion a straddle position will put less pressure on the back, help the lifter remain more upright during the lift, and take away the friction of dragging the bar up the legs. Whichever method you use, it is absolutely critical that you hold the barbell in the dead centre of the bar; even a few millimetres off centre can cause the bar to tilt forward or backward when lifting and produce a failed lift as one end touches the ground. Check the balance of the bar carefully on your warm-up lifts so as not to lose balance on the heavier lifts.

Before beginning the lift, be sure that the centre is positioned directly under your hips on the straddle, or between your feet on the traditional deadlift position. The non-lifting hand should be firmly braced and used to push on the knee during the lift. I am not going to tell any of you how to perform a deadlift, but one difference is that you should try not to jerk into the pull with too much force, as this may be too much for the grip to handle. Ease the bar from the floor and then accelerate if possible, keeping the head and chest up and using the hand on the knee as an additional counterforce.

The rules state that upon completion of the lift, the bar must be above the knees and the legs straight. Unlike the standard deadlift, the rules do not state that the lifter has to have his back totally upright, which in some instances due to the lifter's arm and torso length is a physical impossibility.

Obviously all other rules governing a deadlift—one continuous motion, no movement of feet, not lowering the bar until the down signal is given, and then lowering the bar under control—apply.

I hope you have a go at the single-arm deadlift; as Pullum said, it really is one of the most fundamental tests for finding out just how strong you are. If you don't like the answer it gives you, I suggest you do something positive about it. **M**

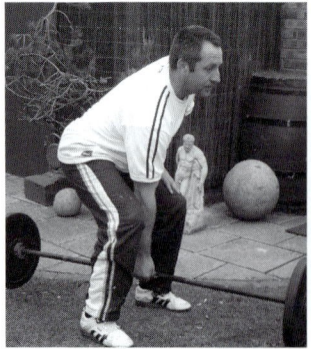

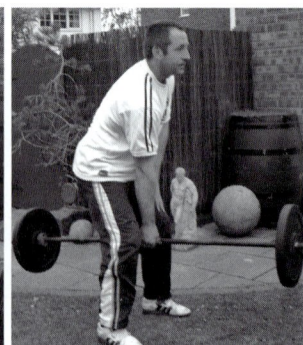

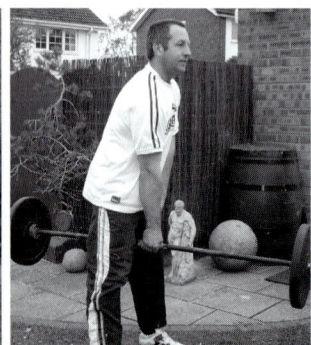

Performing a single-arm deadlift.
Amy Davis photos.

What's in a Bar?

In response to *MILO's* inquiry about Roger's bar and plates, Roger wrote: "Really glad that you picked up on my bar—most people wouldn't have noticed it. It has come to me through various weightlifting friends, and dates back to the 1930s and the Hull–Grimsby area of England. It really has been around the block. I also have some barbell plates from this period from the Camberwell weightlifting club (i.e. W. A. Pullum).

"The knurling has almost been rubbed smooth; it is slightly bent from when one of my weightlifting friends dumped a snatch . . . twice! It is great to squat with, and I have had it loaded to almost 300 kg for partial straddle lifts. The bend makes Olympic style lifts challenging, but then I feel the advantage when I compete on a nice Olympic bar. The plates are just rubber-covered 1"-hole plates to stop them going rusty in my gym.

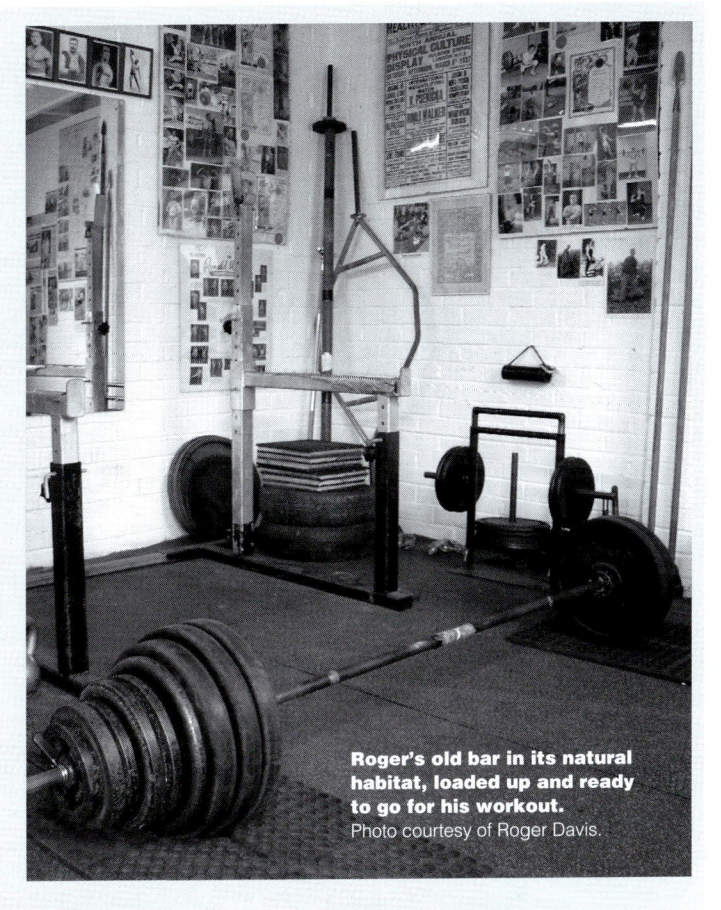

Roger's old bar in its natural habitat, loaded up and ready to go for his workout.
Photo courtesy of Roger Davis.

"Some lifters would just see a knackered, old bent bar that I really should change for a nice shiny one. I see a chain of history going back to the 1930s when lifters were less bothered about equipment and more bothered about strength gains. Off to train in about one-half hour, hoping for a 150-kg front squat and a 195-kg front knuckle deadlift—all on my faithful old bar! I am using both these lifts as a real foundation for my Dinnie Stone attempt in June." **M**

Making Weight:
The Forgotten Discipline

Bill Starr

Author of *The Strongest Shall Survive: Strength Training for Football* and *Defying Gravity*

I was under the impression that the process of dropping bodyweight quickly was common knowledge in the athletic community, but in recent months I have received numerous inquiries on this discipline. Most were from weightlifters, both Olympic and power, but there was also one from a middle-aged gentleman who wanted to shed some unwanted pounds for a class reunion and another from a younger man about to be married.

I think this knowledge has gotten lost for several reasons, the main one being that athletes who have to make weight for contests have started using drugs to aid them in their quest. This became the usual practice in powerlifting: the lifters would use diuretics, either in tablet form or by injection, and then after making weight, they would quickly replace the lost fluids with an I.V. drip. Extreme and somewhat risky to the athlete's health? Yes, but many in that sport are so immersed in the drug culture that a bit more doesn't matter all that much to them.

Then there are the meets where the competitors are allowed to weigh in the day prior to the contest, which kind of negates the idea of making weight altogether—might as well just list the intended bodyweight on the entry form and let it go at that. In addition, a great many lifters never learned how to make weight simply because they didn't have to. This is especially true for those in the heavier classes. Heavyweights have no need to make weight and that also holds true for many who compete in classes at over two hundred pounds.

Finally, those who did regularly lose bodyweight quickly during their competitive days have long since forgotten how they went about it, so this is a short course for those who do not understand exactly how to drop excess bodyweight rapidly while still maintaining a high level of strength, and a review for others. It's done naturally and since it's for a short duration, not all that unpleasant, although it can test will power so it is indeed a discipline. Also, many of the principles involved in making weight can be applied to losing unwanted bodyweight over the longer haul.

I had to learn how to make weight from the very beginning. For the first nine years that I competed in Olympic-style weightlifting, I was a light heavyweight. At that time, the limit was 181-3/4 lb. Early on, I figured out that I could train harder and recover faster when I was a bit heavier, so my bodyweight for training was usually in the 185–186-lb. range—anything higher than that made making weight for a contest a real ordeal. Following a strict, low-carb diet isn't high on the preferred list for any strength athlete.

Making weight wasn't a problem if I knew far enough in advance to make the necessary changes in my diet. However, in the 1950s and 1960s, information wasn't nearly so swift as it is today. There were no e-mails, faxes, or notices on the Internet; it was strictly snail mail.

The procedure went along these lines: I would scan through *Strength & Health* and *Lifting News* for notices of upcoming meets; when I found one which was within driving distance, I would write the meet director, requesting an entry form. Typically, the form would get to me only a few days before the deadline, which meant I had only four or five days to drop my extra weight. I had already started to lower it, but I never really put things into high gear until I knew for certain that I was going to the meet.

Having short notice also happened frequently when I was at the York Barbell Club. There were so many contests available on the East Coast that the lifters tended to forget about them, always looking ahead to the Senior Nationals. It was not uncommon for Hoffman to tell a lifter on Friday that he expected him to lift in a contest on Saturday which he had intended to skip. Bob did this to me just before the Delaware Open. I protested that I had trained heavy on Thursday and wasn't the least bit prepared. The meet in Wilmington always drew some top competitors and I certainly didn't want to get hammered by them only a few months away from the Nationals. It never worked. Bob would say, "Just make it a training session. We need your points for the team title." There wasn't a way out except to say I was injured, but he already knew better so I had to put my emergency make-weight plan into action. I'll touch on that later.

> THE FIRST THING TO KNOW IS THAT CARBOHYDRATES ARE YOUR MAIN ADVERSARY WHEN YOU'RE TRYING TO LOSE BODYWEIGHT . . .

Currently, lifters have plenty of prior notification about upcoming contests, so I'll begin the process two weeks out. With this much time, losing the unwanted bodyweight can be done gradually and when done right, there will be no or minimal effect on overall strength.

The first thing to know is that carbohydrates are your main adversary when you're trying to lose bodyweight, either for an athletic event or in everyday life. Nutritionists have known this for a very long time. Adelle Davis, among others, wrote about it in her classic *Let's Eat Right to Stay Fit* in 1954. The huge influx of new-wave diets and fads in nutrition have since muddied the waters so much that the basic facts have gotten lost in the shuffle.

Here's why your primary focus must be on carbs when trying to lower your bodyweight. What an athlete wants to get rid of when he drops bodyweight is fat and water. At the same time, he wants to retain as much muscle as possible for obvious reasons—so fat and water have to go. Fat first, and then water at the very end of the cycle.

The body is designed to utilize fat. So important is this process that every hormone in our bodies, except insulin, strives to release fat from fatty tissues to be used for energy and rebuilding other cells. Insulin, in contrast, works to put fat into storage. How much insulin we have in our blood is directly linked to our carbohydrate content. This means that the more carbs we ingest, and the easier they are to ingest, the greater the amount of insulin present to do its job. The insulin signals our fat cells to accumulate fat and if the carbs continue to pour in, the insulin levels stay elevated and the fat stays locked in the fatty tissue cells.

It's necessary to understand that we must eat carbs to gather excessive fat in our tissues. The enzyme needed to store fat is alpha glycerol phosphate and it can only be obtained from carbs. This enzyme locks the fat in the cells in such a manner that it can't slip out through the membranes into the blood stream. Therefore, the more carbs we eat the more fat we store. Conversely, fewer carbs equal less fat.

Knowing this, the athlete who wants to lose bodyweight has to begin to lower his carbohydrate intake. With ample notice, this can be accomplished gradually and was the method used by nearly everyone in the athletic community. While bodybuilders seldom had to make weight *per se*, they needed to shed pounds in order to highlight their various body parts. And since most weren't concerned about losing strength, they started dropping weight three or four weeks before a contest. I knew some who were able to drop twenty pounds and would come to the show lean and muscular.

Weightlifters faced a slightly different problem. Their sport was all about strength so they had to preserve this while easing their bodyweight down below, or at least to, the competitive limit. Most started two weeks out from a meet. The initial step was not drastic; we cut our carb consumption in half, but didn't alter our diets much at all. We still ate potatoes, bread, vegetables, and fruit and drank juices and milk, but in much smaller portions. It's not that hard—one piece of toast rather than two, half a glass of orange juice rather than a full glass, and so on. We would eat all the protein we wanted—in fact, the more protein the better. Whenever I'm discussing this process, I'm often asked, "What foods are carbohydrates?" The answer: "If it isn't fat or protein, it's a carb." It's that simple.

> THE ANSWER:
> "IF IT ISN'T FAT OR PROTEIN, IT'S A CARB."
> IT'S THAT SIMPLE.

That first week of cutting back on carbs sets the tone for the next week where things get a bit testier in terms of eating. That's why it's good practice to know how to adjust your carb intake throughout the day. Every morning at ten o'clock, a group of lifters would walk from the York Barbell building to the Sunshine Corner, a small café a block away. We'd stoke up on coffee and some would eat a snack in preparation for the upcoming noon workout. Tommy Suggs always had a small hamburger. When he wanted to drop some bodyweight, he ate only half the bun.

Although that doesn't sound like much, and in fact it isn't, over the course of five days those carbs add up. Many of us started following his example and we dubbed them Suggswiches.

The other thing we did during that first week of dropping bodyweight was ceasing all nighttime snacking. Those who have difficulty with this switched from their usual snacks to a protein food or popcorn—both of these are okay. The protein, such as a can of sardines, added to the daily intake of those much-needed nutrients, and the popcorn without salt or butter provided roughage and virtually no carbs.

Also, that last meal of the day was one comprised of a great deal of protein and fewer and fewer carbs, for example a large portion of pork, beef, fish, or chicken with a salad and little or no starches. This diet helped our cause because after eating a meal which is low in carbs, the insulin levels decline. When this happens, fat is released from the fat tissues in the form of fatty acids and they are utilized as fuel—and this is what you want to occur. Another effective way to lower bodyweight, with most of the weight loss being in the form of fat, is to have long periods where insulin levels remain low and the body is able to burn fat for fuel. That low-carb meal doesn't stimulate any significant insulin secretion, so a meal heavy in protein and very low in carbs at six o'clock (then no other food intake other than perhaps a protein snack until seven or eight o'clock the next morning) will go a long way in helping you dump the stored fat.

At the end of that first week I usually lost about three pounds. I could have dropped more but I wanted to retain as much weight as I could since I still had some hard training to do the week following; just as long as I was in reach of my goal I was okay. Losing too much too early isn't a good idea because that will affect your final workouts before the meet.

Checking our bodyweights was almost an obsession when making weight. We stepped on scales three or four times a day if they were available. If I thought I was losing too fast, which often happened in hot weather, I'd drink a protein milkshake or eat a bit more carbohydrates that day.

> CHECKING OUR BODYWEIGHTS WAS ALMOST AN OBSESSION WHEN MAKING WEIGHT.

By Monday of the contest week, I was usually about three pounds over the limit. Like most lifters who trained hard and competed frequently, I carried very little body fat, so dropping those final pounds was the hardest. I eliminated more carbs: no sugar for coffee or tea, no protein shakes because of the milk, fewer fruits and vegetables, and hardly any starches at all. My diet almost entirely revolved around protein foods.

By mid-week, I would restrict my carb intake to no more than 60 grams a day. For those who have never done this, it's tough to do since carbs lurk everywhere. A glass of condensed orange juice will yield right at 50 grams of carbs, so I had to check everything I ate to see if there might be some hidden carbs. What I and most of the other lifters of that era resorted to were high-protein, easy-to-fix staples: tuna and eggs. I'll comment more on these foods shortly.

> I WOULD DRINK AND DRINK, ENJOYING THE FEEL OF COLD WATER
> AS IF I'D WALKED ACROSS THE GOBI DESERT.

If I were still overweight by as much as two pounds on Friday, I began the most irritating part of dropping weight: cutting out fluids for 24 hours before weigh-in. The internal organs use on average two pounds of water a day to function properly, so I could lose the necessary extra pounds without eating less. This was when discipline was critical. Not being able to drink is nerve-wracking because there are constant reminders in the form of advertisements on TV and billboards promoting thirst-quenching paradise. The only water I drank during that period was enough to swallow my supplements. It was such a relief when I finally made weight. I would drink and drink, enjoying the feel of cold water as if I'd walked across the Gobi Desert. Heck, the lifting was a lark compared to making weight.

While I was eliminating carbs and restricting fluids, I was also loading up on nutritional supplements to take the place of those I was missing from eating fewer carbohydrates. Since carbs supply about half of the energy needs for most people, if they are not replaced, there's no way for them to do anything very physical—and lifting weights is extremely physical. I used a combination of supplements: wheat germ oil, liver tablets, and vitamin B-12, along with a lot of extra vitamin C, E, A, and D, and multiple minerals. For those who can't find liver tablets, use a high potency B-complex vitamin. Liver tablets are superior to the B tablets because they are in a natural balance and they also contain a lot of other vitamins and amino acids. The Bs help you utilize more of the foods you eat and convert it to energy. B-12 is another energizer and we used the injectable form—a couple of shots during the last week of making weight and another the morning of the contest. Should you not be able to get that form of the vitamin, use sublingual tablets. They aren't quite so effective, but they do work.

Minerals are critical when losing weight rather rapidly. Minerals perform many functions that enable the body to operate at maximum capacity. Without an adequate supply, for instance, muscles can't contract properly—not a good deal for a strength athlete. The wheat germ oil was a big plus in giving us the energy we needed coming down the home stretch. Hoffman manufactured and sold a product call Energol, a combination of fish, rice, and wheat germ oil. Dr. John Ziegler told us that wheat germ alone was far superior to the mixture so that's what we used. Dick "Smitty" Smith would set aside bottles of wheat germ oil before it was turned into Energol and we would use those as we dropped bodyweight. It gave us a huge energy boost, which was greatly needed at that time.

Back to eggs and tuna: for the majority of weightlifters and bodybuilders these were the two most important foods when making weight. In some cases, the athlete lived on tuna, eggs, milk and supplements in the final two weeks before a contest. It was not unusual for a contestant to have eggs for breakfast, two cans of tuna for lunch and another two cans for supper. In between, he would eat hard-boiled eggs. I knew a couple of bodybuilders who devoured three dozen hard-boiled eggs a day to keep a positive nitrogen balance—strange, but true.

That was then. Sadly, things have changed in terms of tuna—our friend and standby for when weight needs to be lost. It is no longer wise to ingest large quantities of tuna, or any large fish for that matter. In the last couple of decades, the amount of methylmercury, the organic kind of mercury that contaminates fish and accumulates in humans and other wildlife, has increased exponentially. This very harmful form of mercury comes from coal-fired power plants and affects fish in lakes, rivers, ponds, and streams, and eventually finds its way to oceans around the world. Methylmercury can have an adverse effect on the central nervous system and can contribute to heart disease, high blood pressure, and infertility.

The larger the fish, the more mercury it contains. In addition, waters across the U.S. have been found to contain a variety of prescription drugs, from antidepressants to birth control pills. There are other problems in this regard, but you get my point. You can no longer afford to gorge on tuna; rather, you should select smaller fish, such as sardines and tilapia, or eat much smaller portions of other types. Even while this information is public knowledge, the seafood industry, backed by a wealthy lobby, still encourages everyone to eat two portions of fish a week. It's no longer smart. If you're worried about not getting enough omega fatty acids, buy a supplement—there are certainly enough of them on the market.

Eggs, on the other hand, have been getting a lot of bad press in recent years, mostly because they contain cholesterol. For the record: eggs are the perfect food, and are the standard by which all other foods are compared. They have the highest biological value of any food, with 93.7% as compared to 84.5% for whole milk, 76% for fish, and 74.3% for meat. Since cholesterol is in the yolk, it became fashionable to only eat the whites—utterly stupid. What most people do not realize is that the yolk contains over half of the protein in an egg, and unlike the whites, they have all the essential amino acids, including three sulfur-based amino acids—cysteine, cystine, and methionine—which are very difficult to find in other foods.

> FOR THE RECORD: EGGS ARE THE PERFECT FOOD, AND ARE THE STANDARD BY WHICH ALL OTHER FOODS ARE COMPARED.

As for cholesterol—rather than being a negative, it's definitely a positive. Our bodies have to have cholesterol. It's essential to our nervous system and is an integral factor for producing sex hormones, among other things. The main point to remember in regard to cholesterol is that eggs also contain lecithin. When there is too much cholesterol in the system, lecithin helps remove it. There is a natural balance between cholesterol and lecithin in eggs. Also know that if cholesterol is not ingested, the body manufactures it and that form is harder to get rid of.

What I'm saying is that when you're cutting back your bodyweight, eat all the eggs you want but be conservative with your fish intake. If you desire more protein, you have a wide range of excellent choices.

This plan works well if you happen to be in full control of the situation; however, that's not always possible. For example, when we drove long distances or flew to a contest, there was no easy way to monitor our bodyweights. Also, not every scale was certified, especially at smaller meets. While you may have been at, or under, the required weight when you left home, you'd find that you were a pound over on the official scales.

Aaargh! That's when you have to pull out the emergency measures, which I've done countless times. If the meet site was a YMCA, they usually had a sauna—that worked. So did turning on hot water in all the showers in a bay and sweating for twenty minutes. In the event neither was available, even more creative measures had to be employed. At a meet in Pittsburgh where there were no showers or sauna, I put on sweats, wrapped a towel around my head and neck and drove in a Volkswagen with the heater on high for half an hour to shed those last few ounces. I even heard of a weightlifter at an international meet who shaved off all the hair on his body to get under the weight limit.

And, of course, every lifter did his best to outwit the scale. Most scales were the kind found in doctors' offices. We would move around on the plate searching for the soft spot—that place where the weight changed just a tad. It might be near the front or back, or off to one side, but nearly every scale had one. Once someone discovered it, he passed the info on to others, except to the competitors who were jerks—they were left to their own devices. While being weighed in, the lifter would either stand on the soft spot or put all his weight on one foot without being too obvious about it.

There were other ploys, such as placing a toothpick or match under the plate. The trouble with that scheme was the object had to be removed after the lifter was weighed in and there was a risk of the official noticing this unusual move. The neatest trick was devised by Bobby Hise, who was devious by nature. He would stick a small wad of chewing gum on the little piece of metal that slid on the railing until it balanced. When placed just right it would alter the outcome considerably, by as much as two pounds. Once the weight was recorded by the official, he would flip the metal backward and remove the gum in a quick, nonchalant fashion. Of course, none of these sneaky maneuvers can be done with the modern, computerized scales, but I wouldn't be surprised to learn of other gimmicks being used to beat them to make weight.

I always made weight. Some weigh-ins were easy, some were miserably hard. The absolute worst was when I entered the Junior National Powerlifting Championships in Patterson, New Jersey. I wasn't really interested in the power

> AAARGH! THAT'S WHEN YOU HAVE TO PULL OUT THE EMERGENCY MEASURES, WHICH I'VE DONE COUNTLESS TIMES.

> FIVE MINUTES BEFORE THE DEADLINE I MADE WEIGHT, BUT I WAS TOO EXHAUSTED AND WEAK TO POST ANY DECENT LIFTS.

lifts, but it was a great opportunity for Tommy Suggs and me to party on the Jersey shore on York Barbell expense money. Tommy wasn't competing; he was going to coach me during the meet. After checking in, we shot down to Seaside Heights and did some serious partying, consuming lots of food and wine. I was going to lift in the 198-lb. class and wasn't too concerned about making weight—that was until I stepped on a scale around midnight and in dismay discovered that I weighed 208 lb. I was just under 200 lb. when I left York—how in the world did I gain that much? Tommy reminded me that we had been eating and drinking in mass quantities ever since we got to the shore.

I had exactly twelve hours to lose ten pounds. It was midsummer, which helped. I slept wrapped in blankets, bundled up on the drive back to Patterson, stayed under hot showers for an hour, and used the bathroom as often as possible. All the while, I never ate a bite or drank anything. Five minutes before the deadline I made weight, but I was too exhausted and weak to post any decent lifts. Losing that much weight that fast isn't very smart. There's no way an athlete can perform at his best under those conditions. Over the course of two weeks, it would have been rather easy. I believe that no athlete in any sport should try to lose more than 5% of his bodyweight over a two-week period in preparation for a competition. If you need to lose more than 5%, move into the higher division.

The ideas that I've presented for losing weight and maintaining strength are the same as those used by lifters and bodybuilders in the fifties and sixties. This period was well over a decade before Dr. Atkins came out with his monster bestseller *The Diet Revolution*, which recommends the same approach to losing weight.

The principles work for making weight for athletic events and they're also most useful for anyone wanting to lose some unwanted pounds. For the former, it's a short concentrated effort; for the latter, it's a much longer, less-severe process that may eventually become a part of one's lifestyle. **M**

> THE PRINCIPLES WORK FOR MAKING WEIGHT FOR ATHLETIC EVENTS AND THEY'RE ALSO MOST USEFUL FOR ANYONE WANTING TO LOSE SOME UNWANTED POUNDS.

Strength Skills: Lifting Hard and Heavy

Dr. Ken E. Leistner
Chiropractor

There are woefully few good books about strength training, weightlifting, powerlifting, strongman activities, and any other subject remotely related to getting muscularly larger and stronger. The scientific texts specifically about human physiology, kinesiology, biomechanics, neurology, and gross anatomy—the subjects that do in fact directly concern themselves with training for strength activities—are numerous, accurate, and extraordinarily useful, even for those without a post-high school education. However, once the information in the legitimate scientific texts is collected into the so-called scientific publications on strength training, weightlifting, powerlifting, strongman activities, and any other subject remotely related to getting muscularly larger and stronger, you have little more than what my relatively uneducated father often referred to as "high-falutin' b***-***t."

Almost every study that is sponsored by an entity, especially a commercial entity, has something to prove, something that will benefit its sales or reputation in the industry. There have been attempts at legitimate research but my numerous articles over a number of decades have appropriately derided most of what passes for scientific documentation in our field of interest. My late father-in-law, a highly-respected and internationally-renowned professor and biology researcher at Purdue University, provided ongoing, never-ending, and rather humorous examples of the faulty protocols and procedures that populate the field of exercise science research.

Let me repeat my position as one who has great respect for those who work in our field. We are still very much a cult, a relative few who live, breathe, and are engrossed with the iron sports. Anyone trying to move it forward has me on his side. However, there are few who give a straight story with nothing to sell. I have been friendly with Bill Starr for decades. Bill was a terrific Olympic-style lifter, won acclaim as a powerlifter, placed high in a number of physique contests, and remains the premier writer in the field, hands down. I often read some of his work and think, "Geez, I wish I had written that." Bill's influence, not only through his ubiquitous articles but also through his active coaching, is enormous. One of the very accomplished lifters he has mentored is Mark Rippetoe of Wichita Falls, Texas.

Following in Bill's footsteps, Mark also has a penchant for writing and writing well, including extremely informative books about strength training. One of the best quotes from his book *Strong Enough?* (on the count of three, everyone may yell, "Of course not!") is related to the bench press but is more applicable to training in general. The value of the bench press and the relative usefulness and effectiveness of the overhead press

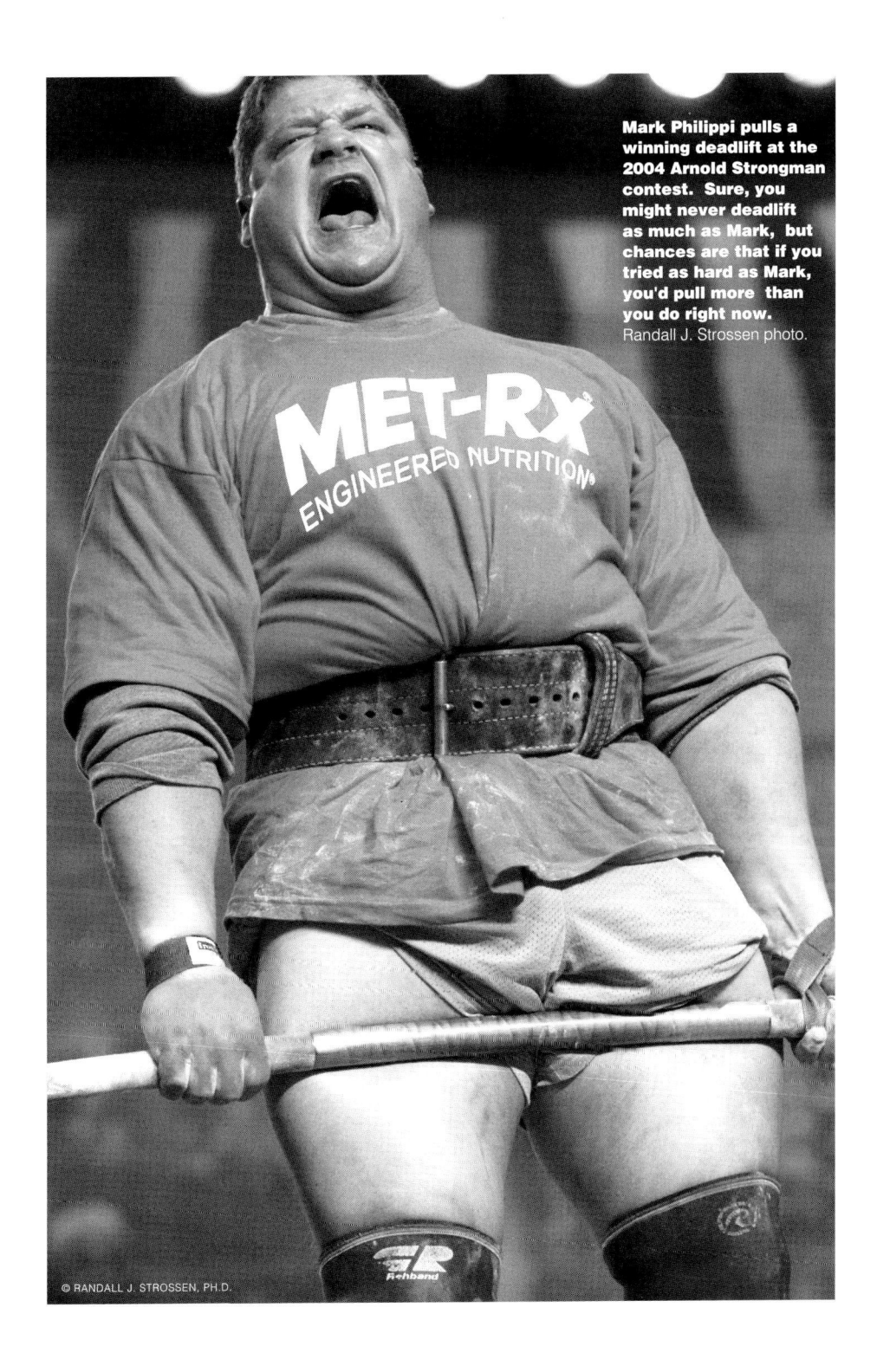

Mark Philippi pulls a winning deadlift at the 2004 Arnold Strongman contest. Sure, you might never deadlift as much as Mark, but chances are that if you tried as hard as Mark, you'd pull more than you do right now.
Randall J. Strossen photo.

versus the bench press have filled many pages in *MILO*, and I am one of the authors who has filled quite a few of them. It's not the bench press, however, that I would like to highlight but instead Mark's well-stated comment about hard work. Quoting Mark on page 36 of *Strong Enough?* with the emphasized part as mine:

"Benching provides hard active work for the chest, shoulders, and arms and isometric work for the forearms, and *it trains novice lifters well in the fundamental skill of pushing on a very heavy load. This last may be its most useful function.* When people first start training, they have no experience with maximal effort. *The vast majority of humans on this planet have never had to push really, really hard on anything,* and that is a skill that should be developed, along with cooking, critical thinking, and interpersonal relations."

Mickey Marotti is the strength and conditioning coordinator for the University of Florida. Prior to joining Urban Meyer's staff, Mickey served under Al Johnson as his assistant at West Virginia University and then as the head strength and conditioning coach at the University of Cincinnati and at the University of Notre Dame. He has developed successful athletes and winning teams at each stop, and his work at Florida was a key ingredient as they approached the national championships for the 2008 season. One of the most important and meaningful statements Mickey made to me years ago, and one that became an article in the previously published *Hard Training Newsletter* by Hammer Strength Company, concerned itself with some of the finishing exercises that Mickey utilized for his football players.

A bit before strongman competition became commonplace, prior to the formation of the various competing organizations, and predating the availability of heavy tires, farmer's walk implements, and super yokes at more than a half-dozen locations in any state, Mickey had his guys pushing trucks, doing farmer's walks, and flipping tires for a two-fold purpose. In addition to enhancing muscular strength and what we can refer to for the sake of simplicity here as muscular endurance, this was a means to force the football players to work hard.

"THE VAST MAJORITY OF HUMANS ON THIS PLANET HAVE NEVER HAD TO PUSH REALLY, REALLY HARD ON ANYTHING . . ."

As Mickey explained to me, unlike the era when we were young, with Mickey being quite a bit younger than I, most teenagers had an after-school and/or weekend job. Mickey and I both had the pleasure of working for our fathers, men who performed manual labor or a trade that required hard, heavy, physical exertion. Mickey's contention, and one I wholeheartedly agreed with, was that young people, including the muscularly large and strong football players he worked with at the highest level of collegiate football, had very little experience performing manual labor or physically demanding work of any kind. Some may have had brief, weeks-long jobs that required some manual effort, but most had not. The majority of the young men under his supervision just did not know how to work hard physically, and the finishing movements provided the opportunity to do so. In combination with intense sets of exercises like squats, deadlifts, overhead presses, and various pulls, many were receiving their first real exposure to hard work, even those coming from a disadvantaged background.

Mark Rippetoe's belief that "The vast majority of humans on this planet have never had to push really, really hard on anything" is in my opinion, an absolute fact. Unfortunately, training hard, working hard at any physically demanding task, and lifting very heavy weights is a learned skill. My statement to new trainees, even those who are already established as successful professional football players, is, "Training hard is a learned skill and like any skill, it becomes better with practice. The more often you train hard, the better you become at training hard, and the workouts that seem so difficult at the beginning stages of our training will cause you to laugh at them in the not-too-distant future when you begin to understand how to train hard." Doing nearly countless repetitions of anything does not necessarily make that activity hard or difficult to complete. One has to learn how to train hard in order to train hard, in a highly intense manner, utilizing most if not all of one's momentary ability to do so on that specific training day.

Olympic-style weightlifting was never an activity I jumped into with both feet. Although I competed a number of times with limited success, I genuinely enjoyed the sport and the company of most of the lifters I trained or competed with. Unlike many self-crowned experts, I know what I don't know and Olympic-style weightlifting is one of those things. However, I do know that a tremendous amount of emphasis and time is spent on technique and a belief that one needs to perfect his technique. As a distant-but-interested observer, I also know that Rippetoe is right: most trainees don't know how to put a truly heavy object overhead or on their backs or take it off of the floor with confidence and a fierce, unyielding commitment to do so. They have never had to work hard or utilize weights that make their proprioceptors go, "Oh boy, this might be a problem."

One of my favorite lifters was David Rigert. I was always attracted to his unbelievable levels of strength as reported in *Strength & Health* magazine and the stories told by the York lifters. I saw films of him in the warm-up room and training hall taken prior to a World Championships, and he was head and shoulders above other lifters in his pound-for-pound ability to move heavy weights. Serge Redding of Belgium was another super-powerful lifter. At the Olympic level at which they both competed, they (obviously) knew proper technique; but from the comments often made by America's best coaches and lifters in my presence, their technique was not as good as many others', even a number of U.S. lifters. However, they easily out-lifted the other lifters who had better technique because they were stronger.

> THEY HAVE NEVER HAD TO WORK HARD OR UTILIZE WEIGHTS THAT MAKE THEIR PROPRIOCEPTORS GO, "OH BOY, THIS MIGHT BE A PROBLEM."

True, one has to know how to lift. But in sports and leisure activities where lifting weights is the primary goal and records, personal or public, are kept as to how much weight is lifted, strength becomes the primary factor. I am not minimizing the skill of lifting a heavy weight or moving a heavy object in any endeavor. Know-how is necessary, but training hard, utilizing heavy weights when doing so, and developing the physical and psychological ability to do so consistently is every bit a set of skills that is not emphasized enough by most modern trainees and coaches. M

The Very Swiss Giant:
Ludwig Lutz

Gherardo Bonini

The famous French professor Edmond Desbonnet considered Apollon and Louis Cyr two demi-gods of strength because they were naturally gifted with super-sized bodies that permitted them to surpass their contemporaries. Another giant, this time from Switzerland, was also a protagonist of fantastic strength feats: Ludwig Lutz.

Lutz was born in Basel, Switzerland on 10 August 1864. The famous German master Siebert recounted that between 16 and 17 years of age, Lutz's weight increased by 25 kg (55 lb.); on the other hand, he soon reached his final height of 1.87 m (6' 2"). He was dedicated to wrestling and gymnastics and joined the Turnverein Burgdorf (Burgdorf's Gymnastic Society). He excelled also in the typical Swiss style of wrestling, the *schwingen*. In successive years, he became a specialist of stone- and iron-ball throwing. During the seasons of 1891 and 1892 he set several throwing records either by running or in the standing position. He launched a

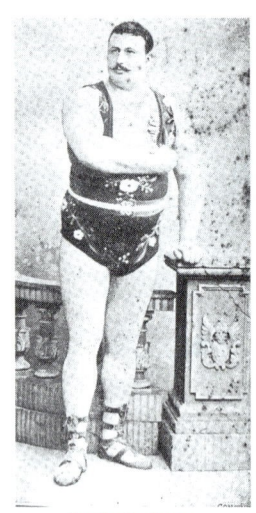

Ludwig Lutz.
Courtesy of Gherardo Bonini.

spherical iron ball of 16 lb. (about 7.25 kg) up to 13.84 m (about 45'), and he was a recognized record-holder for throwing iron balls of 10, 12.70, 15, 19.05 and 25.50 kg (22, 28, 33, 42, and 56 lb.), either by running or in the standing position. With the iron sphere of 25.50 kg (56 lb.) he reached 6.82 m (22') without running and 9.14 m (30') with running.

In the same manner and in the same seasons, he set other records in the specialized areas of stone throwing. The stones were spherical or rectangular. Lutz launched a spherical stone of 45 kg up to 3.70 m (12' 2").

After 1892 he continued to increase in bodyweight. In March 1894 he weighed 134 kg (295 lb.), and at the end of the year 120 kg (265 lb.). In the seasons 1893 and 1894 he dedicated himself to the sport of weightlifting, achieving very good results. He was able to snatch with one hand a dumbbell of 85 kg, which at that time represented a sort of unofficial world record.

Moreover, he was able to hold out horizontally a weight of 40 kg and achieved good performances in the continental two-hands press. Being a colossus, he did not need to indulge in an accentuated back-bend in the final phase of pressing, so his feats had a great value. He pressed in this manner 110 kg for six times in succession, and he then pressed two separate dumbbells of 60 kg each! Probably below his potential was his 93-kg one-hand press in the German style, namely after cleaning with two hands.

In 1896 he transferred to Hamburg, Germany, where he opened a shop for fishing equipment. Around the same period, the famous German expert of strength sports Ferdinand Hüppe (1852–1938) wrote in the Viennese *Allgemeine Sport Zeitung* that Lutz had to be reputed as not the strongest but the most complete athlete of the world. In fact, in spite of his corpulent size, his records in flat races were remarkable. Considering his lifting records, his throwing achievements, and his skill as wrestler and runner, no one in the world could boast a similar curriculum.

At any rate, Lutz remained the best worldwide stone- and iron-ball thrower. In May 1897, during a gymnastic festival in Wädensweil, near Zürich, he exceeded his previous record in stone throwing with 45 kg, reaching 3.90 m (12' 9-1/2"). In the same period; his body measurements were checked again and his weight was 102 kg (225 lb.); his chest 117 cm (46") (not inflated) and 129 cm (51") inflated; his upper arm 45 cm (18"); and the lower arm 38 cm (15"). It has to be said that some of these measurements were very different from those recorded some years before by Siebert.

His best performance in the two-hands jerk was 132 kg, and this record is impressive because he lifted two dumbbells of 66 kg each. Furthermore, according to Siebert, Lutz did not rest the weights on his shoulders as several lifters did, but kept them in suspension. Strangely, using a barbell, Lutz did not obtain better jerks, so it is arguable that his body size and his mental attitude permitted him a higher standard of performance with separate weights. His power, however, was formidable: once, from a seated position, he was able to lift from the ground a dumbbell of 72 kg and to press it correctly with the right hand.

In 1900, Lutz got back sporadically to weightlifting, achieving remarkable results, but afterward his name vanished from the chronicles of the specialized journals. It is a pity that the Swiss sports bibliography has forgotten his name and his achievements, which are not mentioned in the most important Swiss sports books.

> IN FACT, IN SPITE OF HIS CORPULENT SIZE, HIS RECORDS IN FLAT RACES WERE REMARKABLE.

> . . . ONCE, FROM A SEATED POSITION, HE WAS ABLE TO LIFT FROM THE GROUND A DUMBBELL OF 72 KG AND TO PRESS IT CORRECTLY WITH THE RIGHT HAND.

Develop Brute Strength

Steve Justa

Author of *Rock Iron Steel: The Book of Strength*

When little muscles get fatigued, they will shut down your ability to use your big muscles. It's like getting a flat tire on your car—one flat on a car shuts down the whole vehicle. In the words taken from Arthur Saxon, true strength is the ability to lift heavy objects over and over again without becoming tired; or to wrestle a good man in a hard bout for a half hour without becoming unduly fatigued; or to jump on a bike and ride 100 miles without being exhausted at the end of the ride. Gaining strength is the art of building bodily energy along with bone density, ligament and tendon strength, and muscle density. The more energy you build in your body, the greater potential you have to lift heavy objects without being physically drained.

In my mind, strength is the ability to move, lift, or support heavy objects without becoming physically tired. Or to push or pull for a long time on objects that don't move without becoming too tired, as in isometric training. It does not matter how big your muscles are if you haven't got the strength in your joints to control or hold your muscle contractions. Every joint is a weak point that you must strengthen from every angle you can think of. The tendons, ligaments and bones are the supports that guide your muscles, toes, ankles, knees, hips, back, vertebrae, shoulders, elbows, wrists, fingers, and each joint; and the tendons and ligaments that hold these joints together must be dealt with directly and intensely.

For every different lift you do and each different angle in which you move your body, you place different stresses on the various tendons, ligaments and muscles that surround each of these joints. I believe there is coordination from the mind to the nerve to the muscle that is strengthened when you practice different movements. I believe that practicing a variety of lifts develops the nerves more strongly in the direction in which your muscles move in these different lifts.

Arthur Saxon could lift 389 lb. above his head with one arm in the bent press and he weighed only 200 lb. The key to developing super strength at the lightest bodyweight possible is to work as many different lifts as you can. The bent press, to those of you who have never done the lift, is in my opinion one of the hardest lifts ever invented. It takes strength, coordination, supreme concentration, and endurance. The technique itself goes against all your natural instincts in moving your body. It takes years of practice to master, but it works so many different muscles it is worth it. Saxon was putting 385 lb. over his head with one arm at 200 lb. bodyweight—unbelievable.

> **How did Saxon do it at such a light bodyweight? He built up extraordinary endurance strength first of all.**

Tremendous power, strength and endurance come into play when handling such a heavy weight with one arm over your head. How did Saxon do it at such a light bodyweight? He built up extraordinary endurance strength first of all. How did he develop such might at such a light bodyweight? He practiced constantly day in and day out, doing heavy singles for two to three hours a day in the bent press. As I said earlier, the lift works so many different muscles—Saxon was getting a well-rounded workout.

You just can't jump right in and do this regimen; you have to toughen your body slowly. It could take months or even years to get to the point where you can train as hard as Saxon did, day in and day out. Each time he practiced, he'd go to the point where he felt his strength start to drain and then he'd stop. He didn't overtrain, but he pushed his body to the limit every time he did train—that's how you develop super strength. Each time you train, try to do more than you did last time—either more weight, more reps, or more sets—that way you take the guesswork out of things and you are forcing your body to get tougher with your willpower alone. Don't worry about muscle size; always put a premium on bodily energy and endurance.

For all-around super strength, it is best to practice everything: partial movements, full-range movements, one-hand lifts, two-hand lifts, supporting lifts, isometric holds, and pushes or jerks. Do it all—try to work and pull every strip of muscle fiber in every position you can think of. This is how you develop super strength at a light bodyweight, as well as a fantastic build.

Discipline, regularity and consistency are the real keys to the art of developing and building super strength. You have to build the foundation before you can build the house. When starting any new kind of workout or exercise, I have found it usually takes at least a month to start adjusting to it. Be patient and don't get excited; just keep training and before you know it, you'll be breaking through all your sticking points without the use of drugs or having to eat like a horse every day. All you need to develop super strength is a strong will—that's the biggest steroid in the world.

> **All you need to develop super strength is a strong will—that's the biggest steroid in the world.**

I've never, ever, used steroids and at one time or another I've lifted some of the heaviest weights in the world on the lifts I practiced a lot. Don't get worried about not making progress as fast as you think you should; if you just keep training it will all come to you sooner or later.

Almost everyone has basically the same body to work with—it's your mind that will push your body to change. Your will is what you need to build: the stronger your willpower gets, the stronger your body will get. Believe what I say, for I know it is true. You don't need tons of protein, you don't need steroids, you don't need any of that stuff. All you need is willpower and mental drive to push yourself past all your limits. Take it from a pro—what I say is the truth. **M**

2009 European Men's Weightlifting Championships: Newcomers Make Names for Themselves

**Bucharest, Romania
3–13 April 2009**

Per Mattingsdal

EWF Vice President

The 2009 European Senior Weightlifting Championships were held in Bucharest, Romania. The last time Romania hosted a continental championships was a long time ago, in 1972, and after waiting 37 years, the Romanian Weightlifting Federation was once again ready for such a big event. With a personality like Nicu Vlad, Olympic champion 1984, president of the Romanian Weightlifting Federation and also vice-president of the Romanian Olympic Committee, at the wheel of a well-oiled organising committee, the Romanians delivered one of the most successful championships in the EWF's 40-year history. The competition, accommodations, service and logistics were of the highest quality. The EWF's 40th anniversary was celebrated at a worthy gala dinner Sunday evening, with a special commemorative coin designed by the EWF's General Secretary Marino Ercolani Casadei and President Antonio Urso delivered to all the European federations.

This year's European Championships had gathered 143 men and 88 women lifters from 35 countries for the competition. Once again Russia had the best male team with 500 points; Turkey followed close behind in second place at 474 points; and as they did last year, Azerbaijan got third place at 447 points. According to the Sinclair formula, Arakel Mirzoian (ARM), still a junior and winner of the 69-kg category, was the best individual lifter with 452.5 points; the winner of the 105-kg class, Vladimir Smorchkov (RUS), followed in second place with 449.7 points; and the silver medalist in the 69-kg category, Venceslas Dabaya (FRA) was in third place with 448.4 points.

All photos by Randall J. Strossen.

Russia had also the best women's team at 516 points; Turkey was second also among the women with 494 points; while last year's winner, Ukraine, had to be satisfied with third place at 481 points. The competition for the best women ranking was fierce, with only tenths of the Sinclair points separating the three best: Natalia Zabolotnaia (RUS), Oxana Slivenko (RUS), and Nurcan Taylan (TUR).

In early June 2009, the same organising committee will host the 2009 Junior World Championships. When the Romanian Weightlifting Federation at last emerged from the closet, they did it with a vengeance!

56-kg category

Altogether 18 lifters from 14 different countries lined up for the competition of nine medals in the 56-kg class. Had someone predicted a few years ago that the gold and silver medals in the total would go to Belgium and Italy, he would on the spot have been declared out of his mind! But that is what happened this evening when Tom Goegebuer (BEL) went six for six and won the European Championships after tactically perfect lifting, doing 115 kg in the snatch for the gold medal, 137 kg in the clean and jerk for the silver, and a total of 252 kg for the gold. The last time Belgium had a European champion was 40 years ago when the strong Serge Reding won the super heavyweight class in 1969.

Vito Dellino (ITA), weighing exactly the same as Goegebuer (55.71 kg) and winning the silver medal in the total, was a real threat to Goegebuer. He made 109 kg in the snatch for fourth place, started with an easy attempt in the clean and jerk at 135 kg, and continued with a splendid 138 kg in his second try for the gold in that lift. He even had a very narrow miss with 143 kg in his last jerk attempt that would have tied Goegebuer's total. But because Goegebuer reached 252 kg in the total first, Dellino would have needed 144 kg to grab the gold overall.

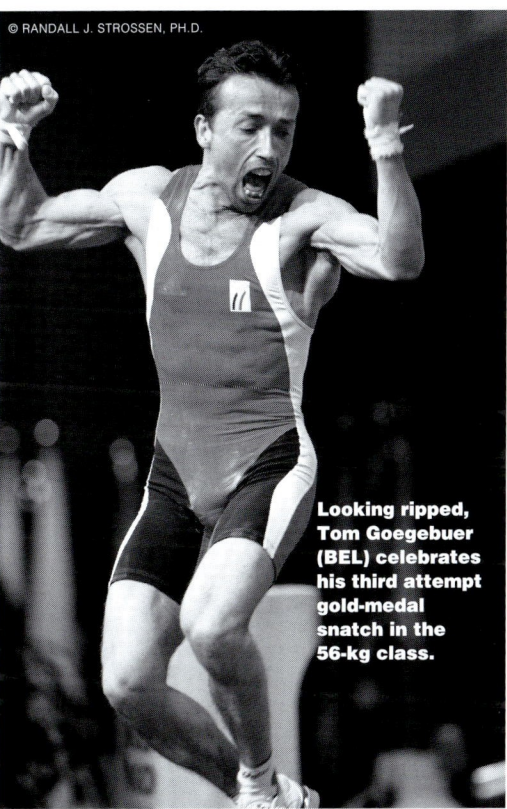

The bronze medal in the total went to an old acquaintance, Igor Grabucea (MDA), with lifts of 110 kg in the snatch for the bronze medal; 136 kg in the clean and jerk, also for bronze; and 246 kg in the total for a third bronze medal.

Looking ripped, Tom Goegebuer (BEL) celebrates his third attempt gold-medal snatch in the 56-kg class.

> IT CAN NOT BE PUT UNDER A CHAIR THAT THE STANDARD OF LIFTING IN EUROPE IN THIS CATEGORY IS NOT SO HIGH AS IT WAS SOME YEARS AGO.

Turkey had 2 lifters in this category. Sedat Artuc ended up with the silver medal (on bodyweight) in the snatch at 110 kg, but could only manage his first attempt in the clean and jerk at 135 kg for fourth place; and his total of 245 kg also gave him a fourth place.

It can not be put under a chair that the standard of lifting in Europe in this category is not so high as it was some years ago. Halil Mutlu's 302-kg total from the European Championships in Trencin 2002 seems unreachable, and the same goes for his world records of 138 kg in the snatch, 168 kg in the clean and jerk, and 305 kg in the total.

62-kg category

The last two years Erol Bilgin (TUR) had to be satisfied with silver medals in the total, but this, the third year, it was time for him to climb to the top of the winner's rostrum three times for the gold in the snatch, jerk and total. In fact he was in a class by himself, making 130 kg and 133 kg in the snatch and 155 kg and 160 kg in the clean and jerk, for a 293-kg total. Bilgin is young at 22 years, so maybe he will be the man to compete with the best lifters from the rest of the world in the future. To be a real threat to the best Chinese lifters, however, he must improve at least 10 kg in each lift.

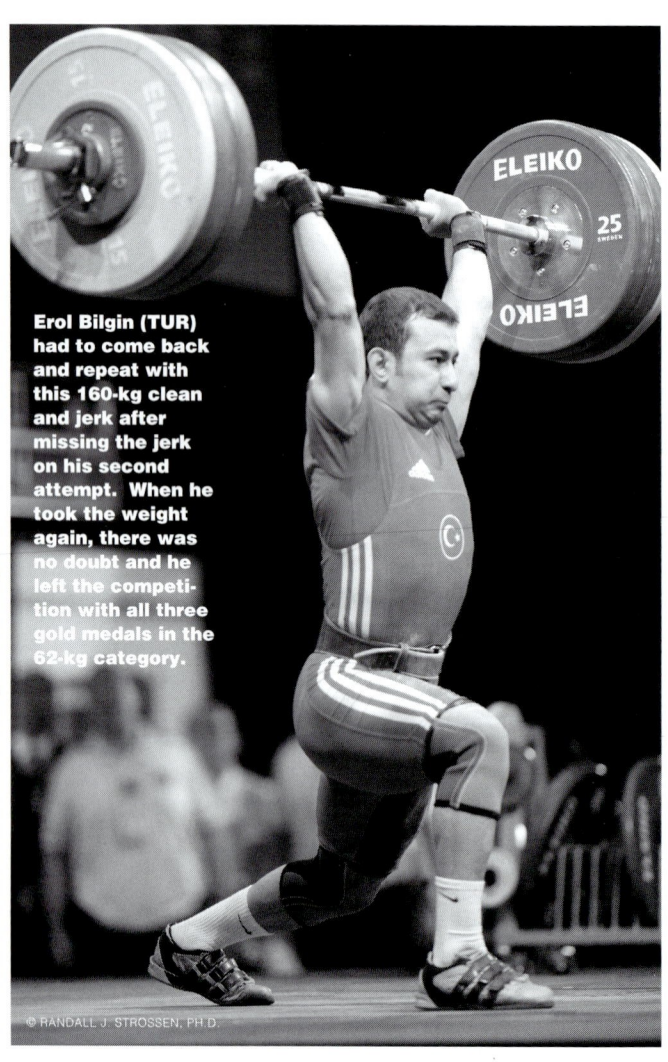

Erol Bilgin (TUR) had to come back and repeat with this 160-kg clean and jerk after missing the jerk on his second attempt. When he took the weight again, there was no doubt and he left the competition with all three gold medals in the 62-kg category.

The battle for second and third place was quite fierce between the junior Dimitris Minasidis (CYP) and Zulfugar Suleymanov (AZE). Minasidis, who competed for the first time in a Senior European Championships, lifted with great self-confidence 125 and 127 kg for the silver medal in the snatch; continued with easy squat jerks of 149 and 152 kg, and ended up with a good one at 157 kg for the bronze medal; he also earned a bronze medal for his 284-kg total. Minasidis also has the qualities of a future champion!

Zulfugar Suleymanov snatched 120 kg for his first attempt and continued with 125 kg in his second for the bronze medal. In the clean and jerk he opened with a good lift at 152 kg. His next attempt at 157 kg was a clear failure, though. For his third attempt he set all his money on an all-out effort at 160 kg for the silver medal in the total. Surely this was his lucky day when, after a great struggle, he got three white lights and was rewarded with the silver medal in the total at 285 kg, 1 kg ahead of Minasidis. He also won the silver medal in the jerk by virtue of his heavier bodyweight than Bilgin.

These 3 lifters were in a class by themselves in this category. All the bomb-outs were also characteristic for this category. In the A-group, 26 of 57 lifts were failures and 3 out of 10 lifters did not get a result in the total.

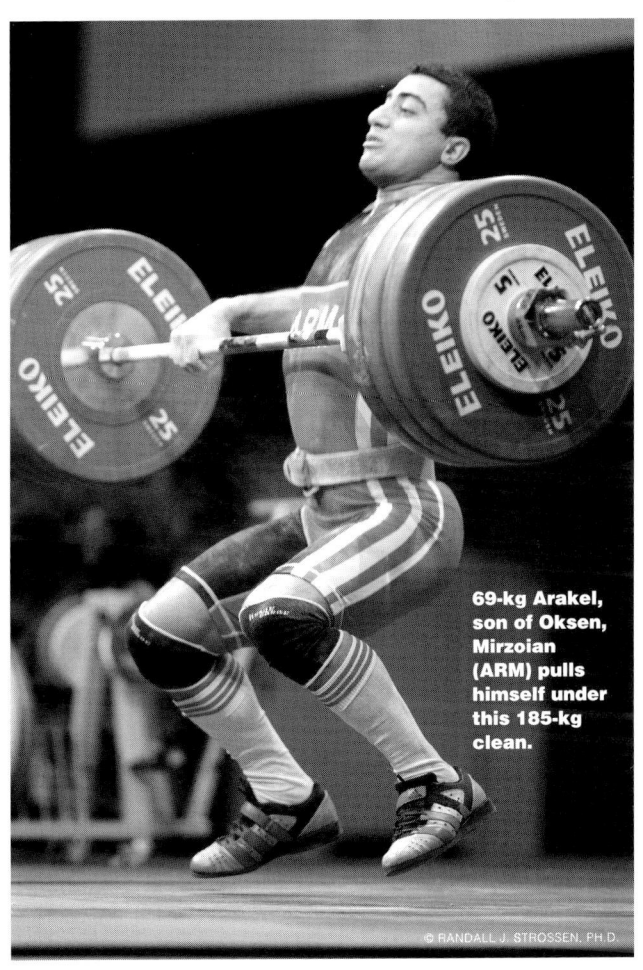

69-kg Arakel, son of Oksen, Mirzoian (ARM) pulls himself under this 185-kg clean.

69-kg category

The third day of the European Championships continued with the 69-kg category, and so far it was the most exciting and competitive. In fact, 4 lifters were fighting for their countries for the most glorious medals: Venceslas Dabaya (FRA), Arakel Mirzoian (ARM), Vladislav Lukanin (RUS), and Afgan Bayramov (AZE).

After a thrilling snatch competition, Arakel Mirzoian was in the driver's seat, winning the gold medal with a perfect snatch of 151 kg. Romania's lifter, Ninel Miculescu, won a popular silver medal at 150 kg. The bodyweight of the lifters then decided the bronze medal position because three lifters snatched 147 kg: Venceslas Dabaya as the lightest won the bronze medal. In fourth place, also at 147 was Afgan Bayramov and with the same result in fifth place was Vladislav Lukanin. Going into the clean and jerk, there was a 4-kg difference between first place and fifth place, so nothing was decided after the first exercise.

Ninel Miculescu did not have the same ability in the jerk as the snatch, and he had to be content with his first attempt at 173 kg for a 323-kg total and fifth place. Of the four remaining stars, Bayramov started the show with a nice first attempt at 175 kg. Lukanin followed at 177 kg for a good lift. Mirzoian came to the platform for an easy 180 kg for a clear lead at 331 kg in the total. Dabaya opened with a good effort at 181 kg. For his second try, Bayramov took 182 kg, reaching a nice total of 329 kg that in the end was fourth place. To surpass him, Lukanin succeeded with a jerk of 183 kg for a 330-kg total and a temporary lead. Then both Dabaya and Mirzoian failed their second attempts at 185 kg. Mirzoian made a strong effort on his last attempt at that weight with a nice jerk at 185 kg, reaching 336 kg in the total and a clear lead. Bayramov failed in his last attempt at 186 kg for the gold medal in the jerk, and then Dabaya made an excellent lift at 186 kg for the gold in the jerk. Lukanin still had a clean and jerk left and he went for an all-out effort at 190 kg for the gold in the total, but that could only be a dead-lift this time.

77-kg category

As in the first three days, the competition in this class also gave birth to a new European champion. The best three lifters from last year's championships did not show up and the stars of the past did not compete. "The times they are a-changin'" is also true in the sport of weightlifting.

> As in the first three days, the competition in this class also gave birth to a new European champion.

We had a fierce fight for the gold medal among the coming stars. The A-group consisted of many newcomers; in fact, 22-year-old Mikalai Charniak (BLR) stole the whole show and captured the gold medal in the total with 344 kg. Behind him by 2 kg followed junior lifter Erkand Qerimaj (ALB), with a 342-kg total for the silver; and the bronze medal was won by newcomer Dmitry Ivanenko (RUS) with 341 kg. It looks as if the federation is preparing new and younger lifters for the 2012 Olympic Games in London.

The competition started with thrilling lifting for the best positions in the snatch. Dmitry Ivanenko had three good lifts at 151, 155, and 156 kg for the gold medal. Mikalai Charniak started with 150 and continued with 155 kg for a success that won him a silver medal on bodyweight. He also had an attempt for the gold medal at 157 kg, but it was too heavy. The bronze medal went to veteran lifter Victor Guman (SVK) with a snatch of 155 kg and Erkand Qerimaj was fourth with 152 kg.

The clean and jerk, as usual, separates the men from the boys and this competition was no different. Mikalai Charniak went three for three, making 183, 187, and 189 kg and reaching a total of 344 kg, which was good for the gold medal. This position was seriously attacked by Erkand Qerimaj, who started with an easy 186 kg in his usual power-jerk style. His next lift, at 190 kg, was performed in same flawless style for a success and the silver medal in the total at 342 kg. Finally, 192 kg was loaded on the bar for his last attempt that would have earned him the gold in the total on bodyweight. Unfortunately today it was too much and he had to be satisfied with the gold medal in the clean and jerk and the silver in the total.

Chalk dust flying, Mikalai Charniak (BLR) hits the bottom with 189 kg on his way to winning the 77-kg crown.

The Polish lifter Piotr Chrusciewicz showed great skill in the clean and jerk. After succeeding with one snatch at 145 kg, he came out like a ghost from a sack and cleaned and jerked 189 kg for the bronze medal on bodyweight.

> AFTER SUCCEEDING WITH ONE SNATCH AT 145 KG, HE CAME OUT LIKE A GHOST FROM A SACK AND CLEANED AND JERKED 189 KG FOR THE BRONZE MEDAL ON BODYWEIGHT.

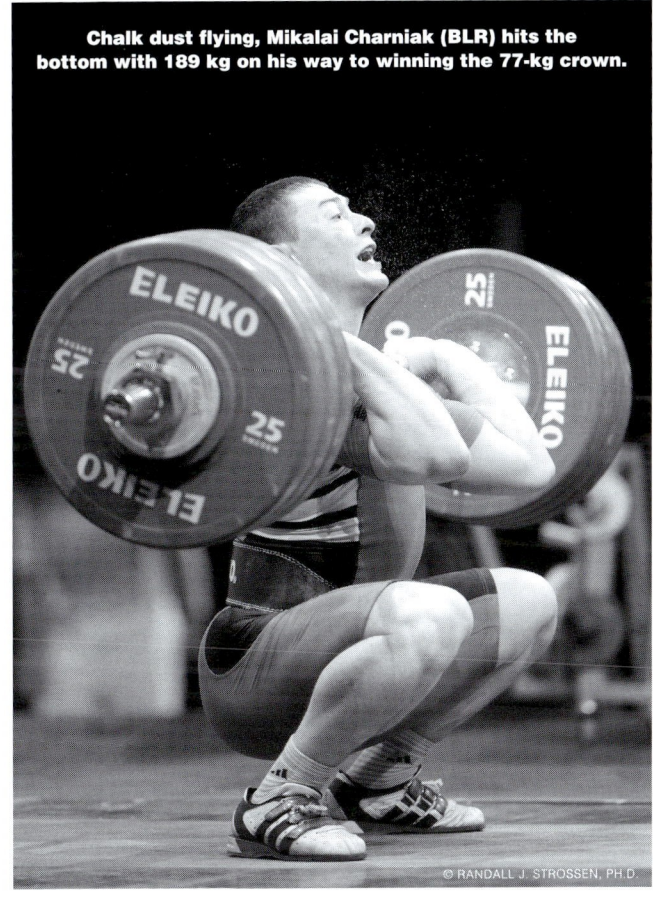

85-kg category

This evening's A-group had a line-up of 11 competitive lifters. Many of them were new faces—only 4 of them from the former Olympic period competed—and all 3 medal winners from 2008 were gone. Twenty-three-year-old Aleksey Yufkin (RUS), bronze medal winner in last year's championships in the 77-kg category, was in many eyes the favourite. As it turned out, this was the most exciting competition so far in these championships—there was only a 1-kg difference between each of the 4 best lifters in the total at the end, and nothing was settled before the last

Aleksey Yufkin (RUS) stuck this 205-kg jerk, good for the gold medal in the clean and jerk as well as the total in the 85-kg category.

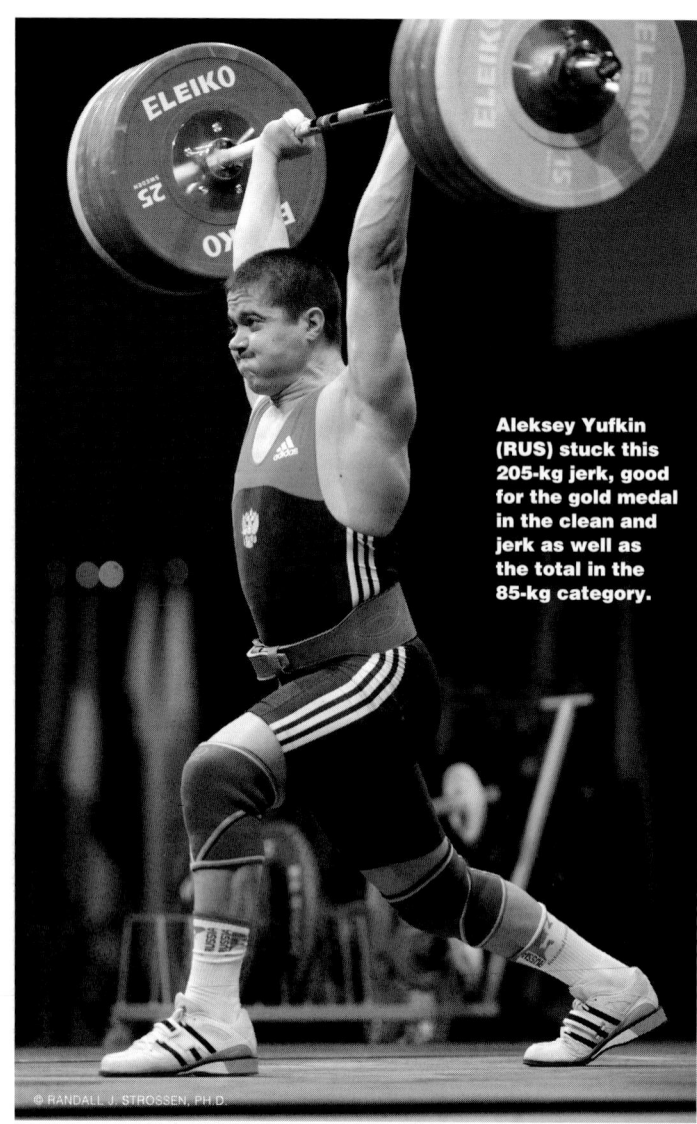

lift was completed. At the victory ceremony no fewer than 6 lifters were lined up on the stage deserving medals.

The favourite, Aleksey Yufkin, had a bad start in the snatch by failing on his first attempt at 158 kg. He asked for an increase of 1 kg to 159 kg for his second attempt for a success. To really stay among the lifters competing for gold in the total, he increased to 164 kg on his third attempt, also for a nice success but only for fifth place in the snatch. Surprise lifter Intigam Zairov (AZE) had the biggest starting weight of 165 kg, no problem. His next attempt, after all the others had finished, at 168 kg was also a success and of course good for the gold medal in the snatch. However, 171 kg on his last attempt was a failure. The silver medal in the snatch was won by junior lifter Adrian Zielinski (POL), who succeeded with a superb lift of 167 kg on his last attempt. One of the other favourites, Mikalai Novikau (BLR), had two flawless snatches at 161 kg and 166 kg for the bronze medal.

Going into the clean and jerks, nothing about further medals was decided. Winner of the snatch Intigam Zairov started with a good effort at 200 kg, for a 368-kg total that in the end took the silver medal. His two attempts at 205 kg were failures. Aleksey Yufkin, as in the snatch, started with a failure in the clean and jerk at 200 kg, but this weight was secured on his second attempt. Of the aspiring winners, Mikalai Novikau started with a nice and good lift at 198 kg; he continued with 201 kg for a success and 367 kg in total, 1 kg behind Zairov's total, but both lifters had more lifts to go. Now it was the time for Aleksey Yufkin to play his last card and he did it well, taking 205 kg on his last attempt for a success and a temporary lead in the total at 369 kg. The clean and jerk specialist, Benjamin Hennequin (FRA), had one more lift to go. He had made nice successes at 200 and 204 kg in his first two attempts, for a 366 kg total and a temporary fourth place. Now he went for what was needed for the gold medal in the total, 207 kg—a lift he failed by a whisker—but the 204-kg jerk gave him a well-deserved silver medal in the clean and jerk.

> . . . NOW HE HAS STARTED EATING CHERRIES AMONG THE SENIORS AS HE WON THE BRONZE MEDAL WITH A LIFT OF 175 KG.

The former superpower in weightlifting, Bulgaria, got a bronze medal in the clean and jerk when talented Plamen Boev succeeded with a nice lift of 203 kg on his last attempt.

94-kg category

The big profile in this category and the winner of the European title for the last three years, Szymon Kolecki (POL), did not compete this year. Only two lifters from last year competed in the A-group: the silver medal winner in Lignano and one of the favourites now, Andrey Demanov (RUS), and Rovshan Fatullayaev (AZE). As in the five preceding classes, for sure we would have a new winner in this category, too. Andrey Demanov started his snatches with a bad first one at 170 kg. He put it into the groove in his second, not quite convincingly, and had to give in on his third try at 175 kg. It was already apparent that his chances for an overall victory were gone. The 170-kg snatch gave him fourth place.

Newcomer Artem Ivanov (UKR) was very impressive, making snatches of 175, 179 and 182 kg for a clear gold medal. Another newcomer, Juergen Spiess (GER), also had his lucky day, making snatches of 170, 175, and 178 kg, good for the silver medal. Nikois Kourtidis (GRE), 23 years old, has been a star since he competed as a youth lifter, and now he has started eating cherries among the seniors as he won the bronze medal with a lift of 175 kg.

Going into the clean and jerk, the chances for a gold medal for Ukraine were very bright. But what happened? Artem Ivanov had no success in all three attempts at fixing the 210-kg overhead that he chose to start with, and he had to say goodbye to the overall victory. Now the road was open for Juergen Spiess. He started with an easy 208 kg and continued with a good second lift at 212 kg, reaching a nice total of 390 kg. This was out of reach for his competitors, and he won well-deserved gold medals in the clean and jerk and total. Nikois Kourtidis started his jerks with a successful 210 kg, good for silver medal in jerk and total thus far. He even tried 216 kg on his two last attempts for victory, but not this day. Andrey Demanov had bad luck with his opener at 210 kg on his first two attempts, but luckily for him, he saved the weight by a whisker on his third attempt and thereby also won the bronze medal both in the jerk and the total.

On the sixth day of the championships we had six new European champions from six different countries. That's very good for the sport of weightlifting!

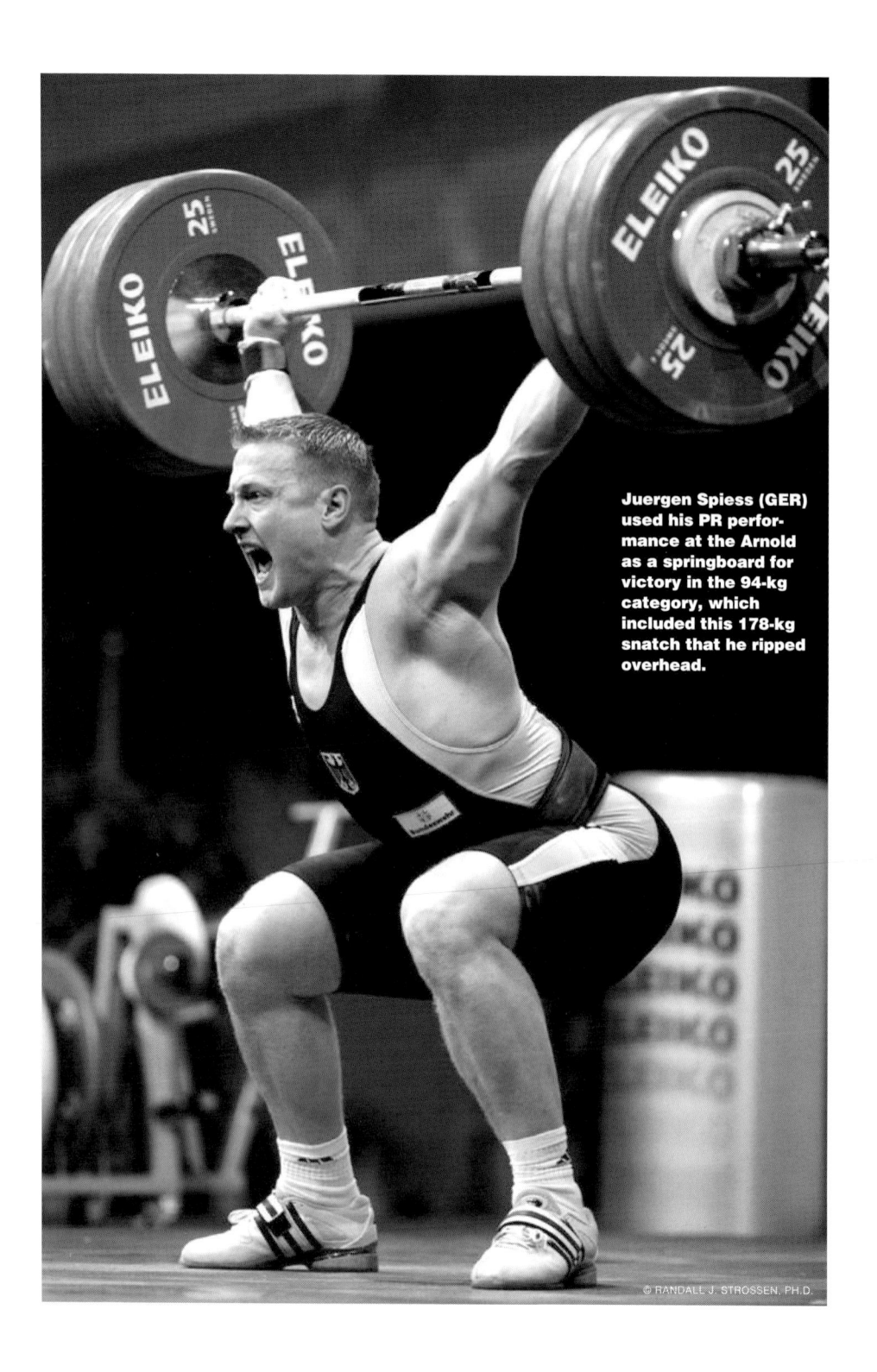

Juergen Spiess (GER) used his PR performance at the Arnold as a springboard for victory in the 94-kg category, which included this 178-kg snatch that he ripped overhead.

105-kg category

Six out of nine lifters in the A-group were newcomers. Robert Dolega (POL), Ramunas Vysniauskas (LTU), and Oleksiy Torokhtiy (UKR) were the only competitors returning from last year's championships.

Vladimir Smorchkov (RUS), European champion from 2005, was one of the biggest favourites, and he did not disappoint his supporters. As the former world-record holder in the snatch, he started his snatches with a nice lift at 185 kg after all his opponents were finished. In his same super style, he snatched 190 kg on his second attempt for the gold medal, but his third attempt at 195 kg was no-go. Roman Konstantinov (RUS), who had moved up from the 94-kg category, excelled in the snatch, making three good lifts at 175, 180, and 183 kg for the silver medal. Ramunas Vysniauskas could only get one good lift, 182 kg, overhead, but he was paid for his effort with a bronze medal. Oleksiy Torokhtiy followed in fourth place on bodyweight with his 181 kg lift, equal to Robert Dolega in fifth place.

Going into the clean and jerk it looked as if the champion from 2005, Vladimir Smorchkov, had the best chances for the gold medal overall. He started with an easy lift at 217 kg, but his second attempt at 221 kg was turned down by the referees. This weight was also used for his third attempt, and making no mistakes this time, he reached a nice total of 411 kg, a clear lead thus far. Oleksiy Torokhtiy started with a modest 213 kg for his first attempt. He continued with a failure at 220 kg on his second attempt, but then made an impressive power jerk at 224 kg for the gold medal in the clean and jerk. His total of 405 kg gave him the silver medal.

Ramunas Vysniauskas, as usual living on the edge, started with 223 kg on his first clean and jerk attempt for a success. With that result he earned the silver in the clean and jerk and his 405-kg total gave him the bronze medal on bodyweight. Roman Konstantinov had a nice opener at 215 kg that gave him a total of 398 kg for fourth place. To conquer the silver medal on bodyweight in the total, he had to lift 222 kg in the jerk. Two times he went for this weight and only missed it by a whisker on his last attempt. Robert Dolega followed in fifth place on bodyweight, also making a 398-kg total via lifts of 181 kg in the snatch and 217 kg in the clean and jerk.

> **Two times he went for this weight and only missed it by a whisker on his last attempt.**

+105-kg category

Eight young, well-built and athletic men lined up for the presentation of the +105-kg A-group. Last year's junior European champion, Evgeny Pisarev (RUS), and Ihor Shymechko (UKR) were top favourites. The old champion, Victors Scerbatihs (LAT), did not enter the championships this year.

Everything was normal in the snatches, Ihor Shymechko started after all the others were finished and made three nice and easy attempts at 195, 200, and 203 kg for a definitive gold medal. Evgeny Pisarev was a little bit disappointing. He started with a good lift of 187 kg, followed with a failure at 193 kg for his second, and succeeded with the same weight on his last attempt for the silver medal, lagging Shymechko by

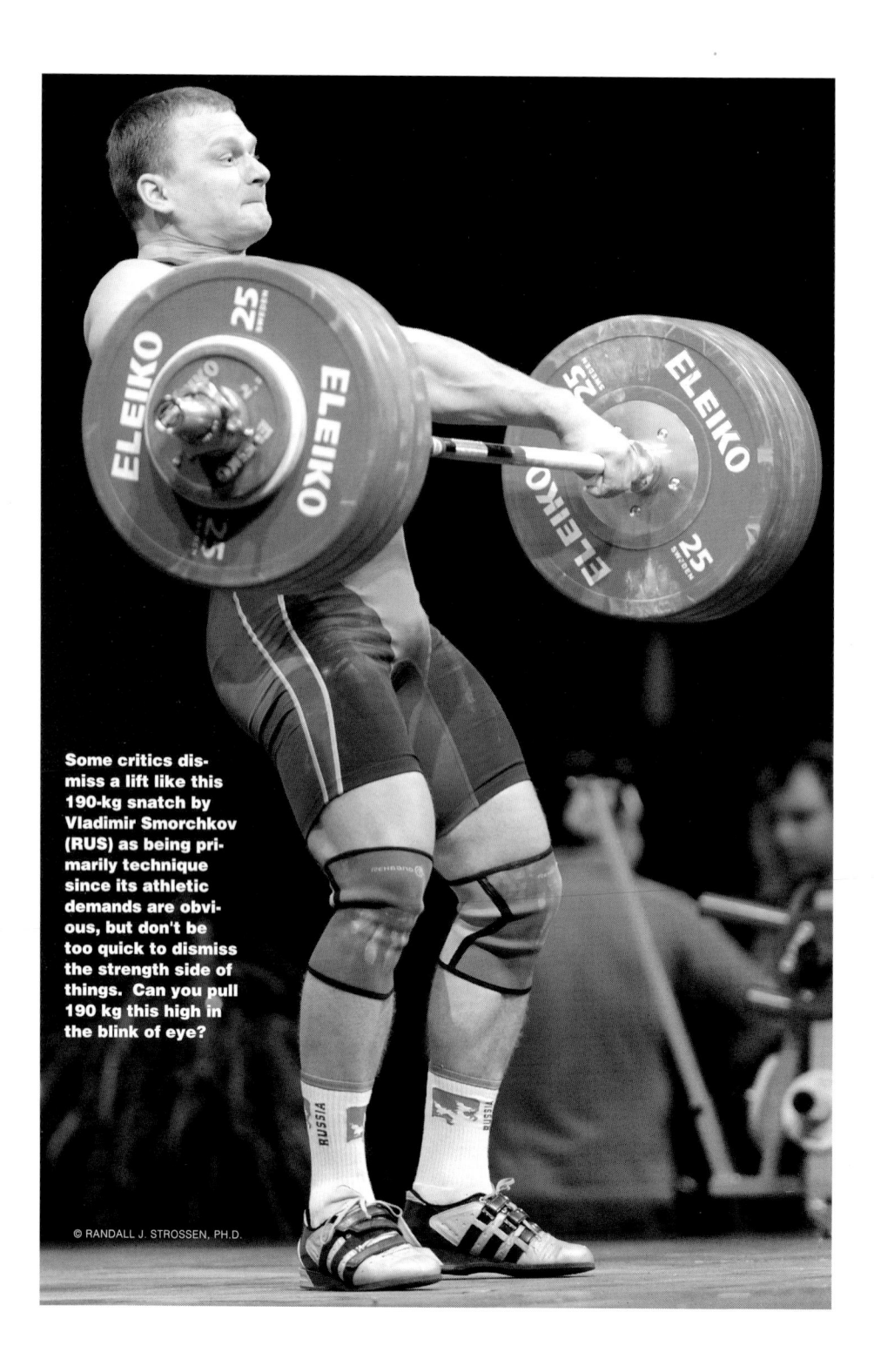

Some critics dismiss a lift like this 190-kg snatch by Vladimir Smorchkov (RUS) as being primarily technique since its athletic demands are obvious, but don't be too quick to dismiss the strength side of things. Can you pull 190 kg this high in the blink of eye?

© RANDALL J. STROSSEN, PH.D.

10 kg. Almir Velagic (GER) was a big surprise and showed that Germany has super heavyweight lifters other than the Olympic champion Matthias Steiner. Velagic made three good lifts at 182, 187, and 190 kg for a well-earned bronze medal. Peter Nagy (HUN) was also a big surprise, making all three lifts at 175, 182 and 188 kg for fourth place in the snatch. The former European junior champion, Igor Lukanin (RUS), disappointed all his fans by failing to snatch 185 kg.

The bad luck followed Lukanin into the clean and jerk when he could not handle 220 kg in any of his attempts. His ill fortune this time was making six-for-six failures, not usual for Russian lifters.

Of the big three names, Velagic started the clean and jerk with a good lift of 222 kg; Shymechko followed with an easy 223 kg; and so did Pisarev by taking 225 kg. For his second attempt, Velagic failed with 227 kg and he chose 228 kg for his last attempt, trying to equal Pisarev's 418-kg total. After a tremendous clean, he jerked the weight to arm's length for the referees' three white lights to the Germans' delight and a bronze medal. Thus far this was also good for the silver medal in the total and so it remained at the end of the competition too.

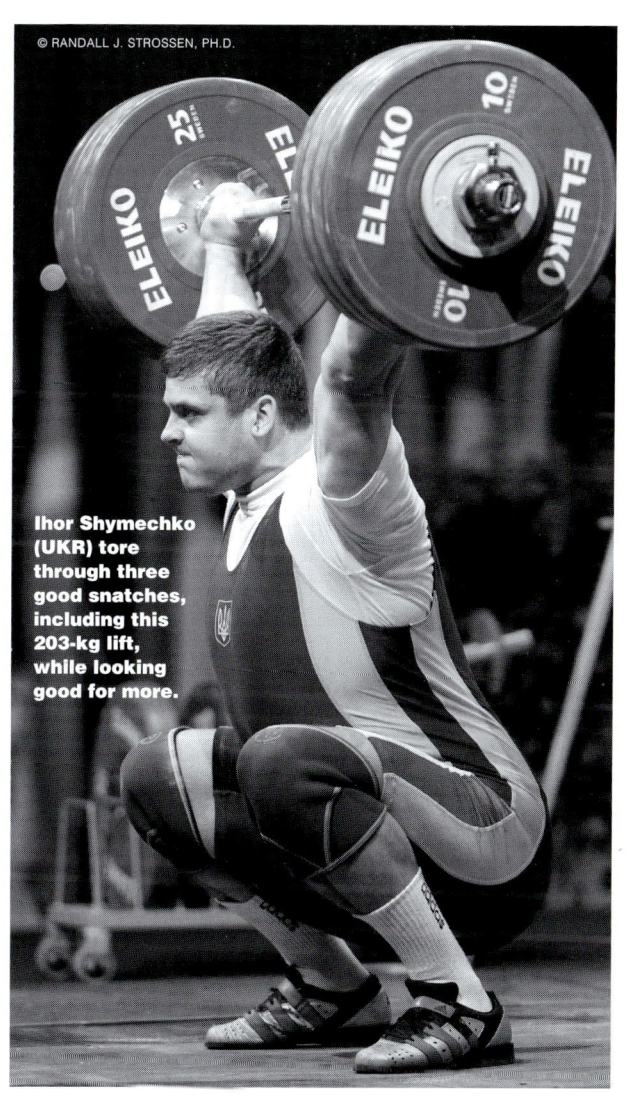

Ihor Shymechko (UKR) tore through three good snatches, including this 203-kg lift, while looking good for more.

AFTER A TREMENDOUS CLEAN, HE JERKED THE WEIGHT TO ARM'S LENGTH FOR THE REFEREE'S THREE WHITE LIGHTS TO THE GERMANS' DELIGHT AND A BRONZE MEDAL.

Shymechko was successful with his second attempt at 230 kg for the gold medal in the jerk and a solid lead in the total at 433 kg. The referees passed two to one Pisarev's second jerk at 231 kg, but this decision was reversed by the jury. Instead of taking the same weight for his last attempt, he increased the weight to 233 kg for a failure in the clean. Shymechko was also unsuccessful with his last attempt at 233 kg. In the meantime, the Polish veteran lifter with the difficult name, Grzegorz Kleszcz, succeeded with a solid clean and jerk of 229 kg for the silver medal in that exercise.

After the lifting was finished eight days later, seven different countries each had a European senior champion, and Russia was the only federation that had two senior champions. ■

2009 European Senior Weightlifting Championships
Bucharest, Romania, April 3-13, 2009

Rank	Name	Nat	BW	Sn	C&J	Total
56 kg						
1	Goegebuer, Tom	BEL	55.71	115	137	252
2	Dellino, Vito	ITA	55.71	109	138	247
3	Grabucea, Igor	MDA	55.64	110	136	246
4	Artuc, Sedat	TUR	55.55	110	135	245
5	Dodoglo, Iurie	MDA	55.49	108	132	240
6	Nazif, Ferdi	BUL	55.97	108	131	239
7	Gulbeyi, Akti	TUR	55.74	107	131	238
8	Olaru, Gabriel	ROU	55.67	100	131	231
62 kg						
1	Bilgin, Erol	TUR	61.70	133	160	293
2	Suleymanov, Zulfugar	AZE	61.75	125	160	285
3	Dimitris, Minasidis	CYP	61.59	127	157	284
4	Sahin, Higazi	TUR	61.54	123	153	276
5	Sirghi, Oleg	MDA	61.04	118	150	268
6	Djelepov, Stoycho	BUL	61.93	120	148	268
7	Wisniewski, Damian	POL	61.46	120	140	260
8	Garcia, Ivan	ESP	61.53	115	140	255
69 kg						
1	Mirzoian, Arakel	ARM	68.33	151	185	336
2	Dabaya, Venceslas	FRA	68.34	147	186	333
3	Lukanin, Vladislav	RUS	68.75	147	183	330
4	Bayramov, Afgan	AZE	68.48	147	182	329
5	Miculescu, Ninel	ROU	68.28	150	173	323
6	Cecil, Ekrem	TUR	68.86	142	173	315
7	Agilli, Ekrem	TUR	68.83	141	165	306
8	Hasanov, Sardar	AZE	67.70	138	165	303
77 kg						
1	Charniak, Mikalai	BLR	76.68	155	189	344
2	Qerimaj, Erkand	ALB	76.45	152	190	342
3	Ivanenko, Dmitry	RUS	76.33	156	185	341
4	Djamilov, Namil	AZE	76.32	151	186	337
5	Chrusciewicz, Piotr	POL	76.71	145	189	334
6	Rosu, Alexandru	ROU	75.50	148	180	328
7	Chykyda, Yurii	UKR	76.56	150	175	325
8	Guman, Viktor	SVK	76.86	155	170	325
85 kg						
1	Yufkin, Aleksy	RUS	84.65	164	205	369
2	Zairov, Intigam	AZE	84.60	168	200	368
3	Novikau, Mikalai	BLR	83.46	166	201	367
4	Hennequin, Benjamin	FRA	84.53	162	204	366
5	Boev, Plamen	BUL	84.81	160	203	363
6	Zielinski, Adrian	POL	84.86	167	196	363
7	Tabaku, Ervis	ALB	84.57	166	196	362
8	Matam Matam, David	FRA	84.74	164	198	362
94 kg						
1	Spiess, Juergen	GER	93.15	178	212	390
2	Kourtidis, Nikois	GRE	93.53	175	210	385
3	Demanov, Andrey	RUS	93.86	170	210	380
4	Fatullayaev, Rovshan	AZE	93.59	161	205	366
5	Gorin, Oleksandr	UKR	92.77	165	200	365
6	Anuskevicius, Donatas	LTU	90.60	161	200	361
7	Cibulka, Lukas	CZE	93.37	144	184	328
8	Hordnes, Per	NOR	93.05	145	181	326
105 kg						
1	Smorchkov, Vladimir	RUS	104.03	190	221	411
2	Torokhtiy, Oleksiy	UKR	104.24	181	224	405
3	Vysniauskas, Ramunas	LTU	104.68	182	223	405
4	Konstantinov, Roman	RUS	100.00	183	215	398
5	Dolega, Robert	POL	104.68	181	217	398
6	Machavariani, Gia	GEO	103.40	180	211	391
7	Babayan, Artur	ARM	104.41	175	207	382
8	Simkus, Modestas	LTU	103.37	180	200	370
105 kg						
1	Shymechko, Ihor	UKR	132.10	203	230	433
2	Velagic, Almir	GER	130.50	190	228	418
3	Pisarev, Evgeny	RUS	137.80	193	225	418
4	Kleszcz, Grzegorz	POL	131.80	182	229	411
5	Nagy, Peter	HUN	142.35	188	220	408
6	Orsag, Jiri	CZE	116.52	175	220	395
7	Sobotka, Petr	CZE	155.06	168	205	373
8	Everi, Antti	FIN	139.05	160	198	358

Advanced Shock and Variable Method:
Compounding to Maximize Explosive Power-Endurance

Steven Helmicki

Author of *The Art of the Neck: Training for Distortion* and *Primordial Strength System*

"Opportunity for advancement always is available for those who remain unattached to convention and limitation, approaching intuitively."

"**E**xplosive strength—neuro-muscular tension in the shortest time possible and quickly bringing the working force to a maximum—is developed in exercises executed with maximal acceleration, at maximal tempo, i.e. under such conditions where the combination of strong tension and speed qualities are required." (Verkhoshansky, 1977)

Everyone recognizes these elements—form perfection, leverage intimacy, tactile education in the various lifts, and enough visible hypertrophy to withstand shock—as all being integral to the foundation of athletic strength training. But the real work begins when the formation of explosive power—and the endurance of it—take center stage. Uninterrupted super compensation within heavy workloads is the goal. Explosive power-endurance is the key to any sport requiring continuous bursts of 60 m or less with short rest periods. Moving within these parameters is often misidentified as speed, but speed does not kick in until post-60 m.

Quickness and acceleration are explosive power-based. Training this way also maximizes type II B muscle-fiber development and in addition to producing astounding quickness, the resulting hypertrophy is significant enough to call for pediatricians to drug test because they state these gains cannot be made naturally. Well, they can—and they will continue to be demonstrated over prolonged periods and across all sports requiring explosive power repeatability.

> QUICKNESS AND ACCELERATION ARE EXPLOSIVE POWER-BASED.

When I adopted the belief that explosive power-endurance should be the foundation and key focus of athletic training after the formative stages listed above, I committed to digesting and re-defining the shock and variable methods to develop this power. Through complexes that continuously evolve, we have been able to produce collegiate athletes who, according to the coaches' reports, are a year or more ahead of schedule in development.

One of our high school programs was not scored against at home and won the ESPN Rivalry Game, and the other program shut out every league opponent in football. The quickness is recognized immediately.

I will share a glimpse of our unique style that produces dominant athletic performances.

"Available data shows that speed of movement is enhanced to a large degree by the variable method [when] putting a shot 'fresh' from the muscular sensation obtained from putting a lighter apparatus." (Verkhoshansky, 1977)

Perform all six complexes one after the other in each training session, three days per week:

Complex 1

Do this circuit non-stop, one exercise immediately after another; go 6 times through with maximum velocity:

• 95-lb. trap bar	x 1
• 10-in. box jump w/ 12-kg kettlebell	x 1
• 12-in. box squat w/ 135 lb.	x 1
• average band# attached pin squat set to half-squat position	x 1
• load until form break or miss on the pin squat immediately followed by	50–90-lb. jumps
• first two ballistic steps out of game stance with average band attached to the waist	

All other resistance stays the same.

Rest/forced hydration	1.5 min.
• 106-lb. kettlebell deadlifts	x 15

bands are Jump Stretch-type resistance bands
* substitute a barbell or dumbbells if you do not have a Sorinex Landmine

Complex 2

Do this circuit non-stop, one exercise immediately after another; go 4 times through with maximum velocity:

• 2-kg medicine ball wall throw	x 1
• 12-kg kettlebell overhead press	x 1
• yoke overhead press 185 lb.	x 1
• double 6-lb. shot put thrusts	x 1
• double Landmine* press loaded w/ 25 lb. each	x 1
Rest/forced hydration	2.5 min.
• 106-lb. kettlebell shrugs	5 x 10
• 32-kg kettlebell high pull	5 x 3
• strong band# face pull	x 25

Complex 3

Do this circuit non-stop, one exercise immediately after another; go 4 times through with maximum velocity:

• 8-kg medicine ball smash	x 1
• 20-kg kettlebell bent row	x 1
• 40-kg kettlebell bent row	x 1
Rest/forced hydration	2 min.

Complex 4

Do this circuit non-stop, one exercise immediately after another; go 4 times through with maximum velocity:

8-kg kettlebell curl	x 2
12-kg kettlebell curl	x 2
16-kg kettlebell curl	x 1
Rest/forced hydration	2 min.

Complex 5

Do this circuit non-stop, one exercise immediately after another; go 5 times through with maximum velocity:

• light band# pushdown	x 5
• strong band# pushdown	x 2
Rest/forced hydration	2 min.

Complex 6

Do this circuit non-stop, one exercise immediately after another; go 5 times through with maximum velocity:

• 8-kg kettlebell swing	x 2
• 24-kg kettlebell swing	x 1
Rest/forced hydration	4 min.

bands are Jump Stretch-type resistance bands
* substitute a barbell or dumbbells if you do not have a Sorinex Landmine

The entire body is worked in these three sessions per week. Each session, reduce the rest/hydration period by 5%. Every three to six weeks we flush, performing five basic movements with an empty bar or very light kettlebell for 50 to 100 repetitions. The program lasts for six weeks. *Polski Energii.* M

PRSRT STD
U.S. POSTAGE
PAID
Ann Arbor, MI
48103
Permit No. 87

IRONMIND®
IronMind Enterprises, Inc.
P.O. Box 1228, Nevada City, California 95959
U.S.A.

ADDRESS SERVICE REQUESTED

****************AUTO**ALL FOR ADC 481
KEVIN E. CLARKE
6918 WISNER HWY
TIPTON MI 49287-9797

Working on a Training Bag

Col. (Ret.) Joseph H. Wolfenberger

I am assuming that most of you martial arts practitioners, boxers, wrestlers, and football players have spent some time working on a training or punching bag or tackling dummy (any device about a foot in diameter, four to five feet high and stuffed with foam, water, sand, etc.). If you don't have one, you should be able to find one at a local athletic supply store or on-line at a martial arts equipment supplier.

If you are a martial arts practitioner, you already know that you can practice almost all of your moves—punches, back fists, elbow strikes, kicks—on this device and it doesn't "fight back." If you aren't a martial artist, boxer, wrestler or ex-football player, it shouldn't take too much imagination to devise a program on your own where you punch, jab, throw or kick a training bag to get a good workout.

I suppose the question that some of you would now ask is, "Why do it?" Being a long-time weight trainer and a karate practitioner for several years, I found quite by accident (since I didn't always have a training partner) that working out on a training bag is an excellent way to vary your weight training program and a good antidote when it has gone stale.

By using your imagination, you can devise a training program on a heavy bag where you work your muscles from almost every possible angle—whether it be punching, pulling, striking, blocking, twisting, or kicking. It does take a little will power and creativity, however.

Aside from the all-around physical benefits of heavy bag training, it has been my experience this type of training can build a certain intangible quality which, for lack of a better word, I call mental and physical toughness and improved concentration. Obviously, it's not going to be like having a hard workout against another individual, but you should not underestimate the value of training on a bag or with a tackling dummy I promise you if you go hard on a training bag, you will be sucking air. You may also feel some muscle soreness in places that you haven't felt for awhile.

For bag-training workouts, I use an old tackling dummy inherited from one of my sons. I have some boxing workout gloves that I use to protect my hands, but I sometimes use just a pair of leather work gloves.

I have listed several exercises and techniques that I use, but I urge you to develop your own program based on your individual needs.

Exercises

1. *Reverse punches.* Stand with the legs in a split position, with the hitting hand cocked and the other arm extended. Initiate the movement with a hip turn, forcefully extending the punching

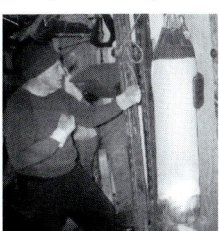

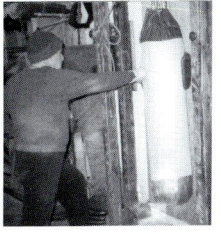

Start and finish positions for reverse punch.
All photos courtesy of Joseph H. Wolfenberger

arm and hand and pulling the other hand to the rear. Repeat for several reps and then go to the other arm.

2. *Back fists.* Stand with one side of the body toward the bag and the (closer) hitting arm in a cocked position across the chest; the non-hitting arm is in a similar position. Initiate the movement by pulling the non-hitting arm back and simultaneously extending the hitting arm and back of the fist forcefully to the bag. Repeat for several reps and go to the other side.

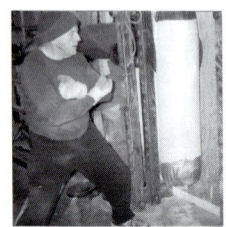

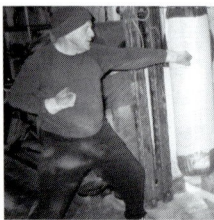

Start and finish positions for back fist.

3. *Combine back fists and reverse punches.* Combine the above two motions into one explosive exercise and repeat for several reps; then go to the other side.

On each of these exercises you can add substantially to the force and power of the movement if you begin each exercise with the knees slightly flexed and forcefully extend them during the execution phase of the movement.

4. *Round house punches.* Stand in the starting position for the reverse punch and keep the hitting arm slightly flexed (bent) at the elbow; forcefully turn the body, pulling the arm into the bag. Repeat for several reps and go to the other side.

5. *Rapid straight punches.* Stand with the feet about shoulder-width apart, facing the bag and with the arms in the cocked position. Punch hard with one arm and then immediately follow with the other arm and back to the first arm, repeating the punching movement as hard and as fast as you can for reps. This one should really make you suck air.

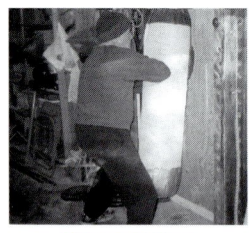

Elbow strikes.

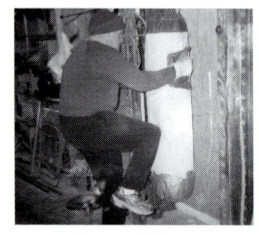

Knee strikes.

6. *Elbow strikes.* Stand close to the bag with one hand behind it and strike the bag hard with the elbow, at the same time pulling the bag toward you with the other hand. Repeat as above.

7. *Knee strikes.* Stand facing the bag with both hands behind it, a little lower than shoulder level. Execute the movement by forcefully raising one knee against the bag and simultaneously pulling down with the hands hard. Repeat for several reps and go to the other knee.

8. *Side kick.* Stand with one side of the body toward the bag about two steps away from it. Execute the movement by quickly sidestepping toward the bag and kicking straight sideways. You can increase the force of your kick by regular practice and by consciously pulling the opposing arm to the rear (e.g. when the right leg is kicking, pull the left arm forcefully to the rear).

These are just samples exercises; I urge you to add your own. Use your imagination and put some effort into it and you'll be surprised by the results and benefits. If you spend some time working on a training bag, you will be able to handle yourself significantly better in a physical encounter against another individual. **M**

The Iron Mine

Associations

The Association of Oldtime Barbell & Strongmen
A not-to-be-missed annual reunion and dinner—coming up, it's on June 13, 2009—for some of the biggest names in the Iron Game. Members receive a very interesting newsletter. Annual donation is $25, payable to AOBS, c/o Artie Drechsler, President, 33-30 – 150th Street, Flushing, NY 11354; email: lifttech@earthlink.net; www.wlinfo.com.

Join USA Weightlifting!
The National Governing Body for the Olympic sport. Go to www.usaweightlifting.org or call 719-866-4508, for news about recent competitions and courses, membership information, local and national events, coaching education, and the newest items available on-line. Membership benefits include participant accident insurance, a subscription to *Weightlifting, USA*, and **super discounts** on airline tickets, hotels, car rentals, and other products and services through our Olympic partnership!

Equipment

York Barbell Club Classic T-Shirts
Available now: 1-800-978-0206. www.oldtimestrongman.com.

Real Wood Strongman Logs
for log pressing. Heavy-duty, sturdy, stellar . . . built to last. www.slatershardware.com; 740-654-2204; Slater's Hardware, steve@slatershardware.com.

IronMind Goods in Germany!
Books, gear, equipment and MORE! www.c·of-c.de, Choice of Champions, Dr. Hermann Korte, Recklinghaeuser Str. 119, 45721 Haltern am See, Germany; e-mail info@k3k.de.

Inch (Replica) Dumbbells in Europe
Top quality and save money on shipping. Please e-mail Nathan Holle for details: nathan.holle@ntlworld.com.

Equipment

Olympic Barbells & Equipment
Tom DiFilippi Sr. (sales rep). 661-723-0614 or tadeagle@hotmail.com.

Strength Equipment/Stone Molds
Nothing but the best strength training/strongman equipment: harnesses, stone molds, kettlebells, books, DVDs and more. www.totalperformancesports.com. 617-387-5998.

Strength Equipment
from the FIRST to close the No. 3 Captains of Crush® Gripper. Custom super-duty racks, benches and selectorized machines by Sorinex. Owned, designed and tested to be virtually bombproof by Richard Sorin. 16 years of experience supplying universities, gyms and serious lifters nationwide. Call and talk with The Grip Man at 877-767-4639, P.O. Box 121, Irmo, SC 29063; visit our website at www.sorinex.com and see our training tips section!

Free Catalog: IronMind Enterprises Tools of the Trade for Serious Strength Athletes
IronMind is the home of Captains of Crush® Grippers, *SUPER SQUATS*, Just Protein®, *MILO*®, the Vulcan Racks II+ System Squat Racks, Strong-Enough Lifting Straps™, and the Draft Horse Pulling Harness™, not to mention the world's leading line of grip tools, a top-quality line of gym equipment, strongman training equipment for the world's strongest men, and books, posters, and DVDs to inform and inspire you to greater success. While we sell plenty of equipment to champion strength athletes around the world, our specialty is the dedicated home trainer—strong guys who train in their garages, basements and backyards. Come take a look at what we have to offer. P.O. Box 1228 , Nevada City, CA 95959 USA; t - 530-272-3579; f – 530-272-3095; website and on-line store: www.ironmind.com; e-mail: sales@ironmind.com.

Equipment

World-class VULKAN Supports
Heavy-duty, high-quality: knee, arm, back, & pants for strongman, powerlifters, heavy events, bodybuilders. Retail & wholesale. www.theweakgeteaten.com.

Finally! Affordable Atlas Stone Molds!
Easy to make, hard to break, heavy-duty poly-Lexan, for time-after-time uses. 8, 10, 12, 14, 16, 18, 20, & 24-inch dia. sizes with complete instructions. We ship internationally. 740-654-2204. www.slatershardware.com, steve@slatershardware.com, or www.totalperformancesports.com, or www.marunde-muscle.com, or www.prowriststraps.com.

CoC Key: From Miles to Mils
Trim that gap (between the handles of your Captains of Crush Grippers) and then make it disappear! The CoC Key will help you unlock your next rounds of PRs, giving you a precise way to gauge your progress. How big was that gap, really? With steps of 2, 4, 6, 8, 10, 12, 14 and 16 mm, the CoC Key will tell you exactly where you are . . . which is the first step to getting where you'd rather be. $9.95 + S&H: $4 USA, US$7 Canada, US$13 all others. Visit our on-line store at www.ironmind.com.

Strong, Pain-Free Hands
In one convenient package: now **three** vital training tools and guide for preventing, reducing, or eliminating hand pain. Kit includes IronMind EGG, Expand-Your-Hand Bands, new Easy Wrist-Relief Soft Weight, and booklet "How to Develop Strong, Pain-Free Hands." $51.85 + S&H: $12 USA, US$18 Canada, US$35 all others. Available in our on-line store at www.ironmind.com, or send payment to IronMind Enterprises, Inc., P.O. Box 1228, Nevada City, CA 95959 USA.

The Iron Mine

Websites, Training Forums

The IronMind News
The Strength World's News Source. Fast. Accurate. Objective. www.ironmind.com.

Sustain Strength & Speed
Battling Ropes: you read about them in *MILO*. Learn more John Brookfield's strength and conditioning system at www.battlingropes.com.

Captains of Crush Grippers Fans
The facts, fiction, myths about Captains of Crush Grippers, and more: training programs, history highlights, gripper glossary, how-tos & FAQs—it's all here. www.captainsofcrushgrippers.com.

PrimordialStrengthSystems.com
Creating the most explosive athletes through the science of persistence.

Strong and Healthy Hands for Everyone
www.strongandhealthyhands.com.

Strengthcoach.tv
For trainees and coaches – advancing the fundamental, creative, and limitless potential of strength development methodology.

Training: Magazines, Books, DVDs

Jerking Routine—For Success
By former national champion & current cert. coach. $19.95 ppd. Send MO to Thomas DiFilippi Sr., PO Box 484, Lancaster, CA 93584.

World Weightlifting
The official magazine of the International Weightlifting Federation; its four issues a year cover contests worldwide. $40/year Europe, $50 elsewhere. World Weightlift-ing, IWF Secretariat, 1146 Budapest, Istvanmezei ut 1-3, Hungary.

Powerlifting USA
Contest results, schedules, training. 12 iss/year; $36.95 US; $96.00 elsewhere. PLUSA, P. O. Box 467, Camarillo, CA 93011.

Starr Novel
The Susquehanna River Hills Chronicles, a novel by Bill Starr. $20 + $6 S&H USA; 1011 Warwick Drive, #3-C, Aberdeen, MD 21001.

Training: Magazines, Books, DVDs

Free Illustrated Catalog!
Books, courses, back-date magazines, out-of-prints, new, etc. Classic how-to training methods and biographies by all the old masters. Buy, sell, trade, collecting over 25 years. Bill Hinbern , 32430-E Cloverdale, Farmington , MI 48336 ; www.superstrengthbooks.com.

***Power Training*—New!**
Looking to improve overall speed, strength, stability, and above all, power? Then, power training—specifically plyometrics and weightlifting—is what you are seeking, and coaching duo Waller & Piper have put it all together in their new training compendium *Power Training*: instruction, technique, exercises, programs, photos, everything needed to guide coaches and lifters through the how-tos. 260 pp. $29.95 plus S&H: $12/US; $18/Can; $35/all others; www.ironmind.com.

Updated! ***Mastery of Hand Strength***
Now with 10% more material and 38 new exercises, all newly-minted material that is typical of John Brookfield's creativity and cutting-edge thinking. If strong hands and mighty wrists appeal to you, this book is your starting point for a world-class grip and lower-arm strength. 144 pp. $19.95 + S&H: $5.00 USA, US$7.00 Can., US$13.00 all others. IronMind Enterprises, www.ironmind.com.

Steve Justa's "High Plains Heavy Metal IronMaster's Bible"
No bull, strength building tips. 20 big pages, big lifts, big poses, over 40 photos. Send $20.00 to Steve Justa, Box 97, Harvard, NE 68944.

Weightlifting Videos
20 high-quality DVDs from every weight class of the 2006 USA W/L Nat. Jr. Champs & Pan-Am Qualifier, $30/session; e-mail WeightliftingVideoDirect@gmail.com for compressed samples or to order.

Denis Reno's Newsletter
The quickest and best way to get Olympic weightlifting results, from local contests to World Championships. $26/year US, $30 Can., $45–$50 others. Denis Reno, 30 Cambria Road, Newton, MA 02165; e-mail: renoswlnl@rcn.com.

Training: Magazines, Books, DVDs

Paul Anderson's Books and Tapes
The Paul Anderson Youth Home offers a free catalog of Paul's books and tapes, as well as the Coleman video on Paul's life. This gives you a unique opportunity to learn from the world's strongest man while helping to support the youth home which Paul Anderson was dedicated to building. For a copy of this catalog, contact: Paul Anderson Youth Home, P. O. Box 525, Vidalia, GA 30475, e-mail: info@payh.org.

***ARM SPORT* Newsletter**
If you're into arm sports, you'd better subscribe to *ARM SPORT*. Results, training, technique, schedules, etc. Four issues a year (US$) $14 US, $16 Can., $28 others to USAA/USWA, Box 746, Billings, MT 59105, 406-245-1560; www.usarmwrestling.com.

Dynamic Duo
These two books, which can be read in either order, give you some powerful psychological tools to harness your mind for success: *IronMind: Stronger Minds, Stronger Bodies* and *Winning Ways: How to Succeed In the Gym and Out* by Randall J. Strossen, Ph.D. are the user manuals that will guide and accelerate your growth. Special pricing for both: $33.90 plus S&H: $10/US; $13/Can; $30/all others. Order from IronMind Enterprises, Inc. via our on-line store at www.ironmind.com.

Defying Gravity
by Bill Starr. Signed. Hard cover $20, soft cover $15 + $4.00 S&H. Bill Starr, 1011 Warwick Drive, #3-C, Aberdeen, MD 21001.

The Iron Mine

Looking to buy or sell? Want to give your upcoming contest an extra boost? Advertise in the Iron Mine. $10 per line per insertion. No display ads, please. All material subject to approval. Send advertising copy or direct questions to: *MILO*, P.O. Box 1228, Nevada City, CA 95959, tel 530-272-3579, fax 530-272-3095, sales@ironmind.com. *We try to screen the advertising, but let the buyer beware.*